DEJA REVIEW™
Microbiology and Immunology

NOTICE

Medicine is an ever-changing science. As new research and clinical experience broaden our knowledge, changes in treatment and drug therapy are required. The authors and the publisher of this work have checked with sources believed to be reliable in their efforts to provide information that is complete and generally in accord with the standards accepted at the time of publication. However, in view of the possibility of human error or changes in medical sciences, neither the authors nor the publisher nor any other party who has been involved in the preparation or publication of this work warrants that the information contained herein is in every respect accurate or complete, and they disclaim all responsibility for any errors or omissions or for the results obtained from use of the information contained in this work. Readers are encouraged to confirm the information contained herein with other sources. For example and in particular, readers are advised to check the product information sheet included in the package of each drug they plan to administer to be certain that the information contained in this work is accurate and that changes have not been made in the recommended dose or in the contraindications for administration. This recommendation is of particular importance in connection with new or infrequently used drugs.

DEJA REVIEW™
Microbiology and Immunology

Third Edition

Eric M. Chen, MD

Bay Imaging Consultants, Inc.
Walnut Creek, California

Joseph J. Chen

University of California, Irvine
School of Medicine
Class of 2020
Irvine, California

New York   Chicago   San Francisco   Athens   London   Madrid
Mexico City   Milan   New Delhi   Singapore   Sydney   Toronto

Deja Review™: Microbiology and Immunology, Third Edition

Copyright © 2020 by McGraw-Hill Education. All rights reserved. Printed in the United States of America. Except as permitted under the United States Copyright Act of 1976, no part of this publication may be reproduced or distributed in any form or by any means, or stored in a data base or retrieval system, without the prior written permission of the publisher.

Previous editions copyright © 2010, 2007 by The McGraw-Hill Companies, Inc.

1 2 3 4 5 6 7 8 9 LCR 24 23 22 21 20

ISBN 978-1-260-44141-3
MHID 1-260-44141-5

This book was set in Palatino by MPS Limited.
The editors were Bob Boehringer and Christina Thomas.
The production supervisor was Catherine Saggese.
Project management was provided by Poonam Bisht, MPS Limited.
This book is printed on acid-free paper.

Library of Congress Cataloging-in-Publication Data

Names: Chen, Eric M., author. | Chen, Joseph, 1993-, author.
Title: Deja review. Microbiology and immunology / Eric M. Chen, Joseph
  Chen.
Other titles: Microbiology and immunology | Deja review.
Description: Third edition. | New York : McGraw-Hill Education, [2020] |
  Series: Deja review | Includes index. | Summary: "This high-yield,
  rapid-fire Q&A book simulates flashcards in a book to help medical
  students review microbiology and immunology for their course exams as
  well as prepare for the USMLE Step 1. It is also a great review for
  students in basic courses in other health-related programs"—Provided
  by publisher.
Identifiers: LCCN 2019047312 | ISBN 9781260441413 (paperback) | ISBN
  9781260441420 (ebook)
Subjects: MESH: Microbiological Phenomena | Immunity | Examination Question
Classification: LCC QR182.55 | NLM QW 18.2 | DDC 616.07/9076—dc23
LC record available at https://lccn.loc.gov/2019047312

McGraw-Hill books are available at special quantity discounts to use as premiums and sales promotions, or for use in corporate training programs. To contact a representative please visit the Contact Us pages at www.mhprofessional.com.

Contents

Student Reviewers

Blake Arthurs
Wayne State University School of Medicine
Class of 2019

Cynthia Wang
Washington University School of Medicine
Class of 2019

Second Edition Contributing Authors

Elysia Alvarez
Medical Student
University of California Irvine School

Nick Boehling
Medical Student
University of California Irvine School

Stephanie Channual
Resident, Department of Radiology
University of California Los Angeles

Keira A. Cohen
Medical Student
University of Pennsylvania School of
   Medicine

Natalie Hoffman
Resident, Department of Family and
   Preventive Medicine
University of California San Diego

Sanjay S. Kasturi, MD
Resident, Division of Urology
University of Pennsylvania

Mara G. Shainheit
Post-Doctoral Fellow
Pathology Department,
Immunology Program
Tufts University School of Medicine

Preface

One of the most important tasks as a medical student in the preclinical years is preparing for the United States Medical Licensing Examination (USMLE) Step 1 exam. Having recently completed the USMLE Step 1 exam, we understand how stressful and daunting it is to learn and retain such a vast amount of knowledge in a short time frame. While everyone studies differently, we believe there are two principles fundamental to any successful study strategy: (1) a solid comprehension of the subjects and (2) repetition of key facts. The Deja Review series is a unique resource designed around these two principles. The series allows you to determine your level of knowledge on the subjects and review the essential facts tested on the USMLE Step 1. We believe this series can help you build a solid foundation that will not only serve you well for achieving your goal score on the USMLE Step 1 but also facilitate a smooth transition into the clinical years of medical school.

ORGANIZATION:

This book covers commonly tested USMLE Step 1 microbiology and immunology topics in a question and answer format. The microbiology material is divided into chapters organized by classes of pathogens and body systems. The immunology material covers basic principles, pathological processes, and laboratory sciences. In this third edition, additional emphasis has been placed on clinical relevance of the topics to better reflect the current trend in the USMLE Step 1.

We believe the question and answer format of this book has several important advantages.

1. It provides a rapid straightforward way to identify and assess your strengths and weaknesses.
2. It serves as a quick, last-minute review of high yield facts.
3. It allows you to efficiently review and commit to memory a large body of information.

At the end of each chapter, you will find clinical vignettes designed to reflect the most common ways high yield pathologies are presented on USMLE Step 1 and other standardized examinations. The questions associated with each clinical vignette are intended to encourage critical thinking in a clinical context. A mastery of the concepts in the clinical vignettes will help you on standardized exams and prepare you for the clinical years of medical school and beyond.

HOW TO USE THIS BOOK:

This text was assembled with the intent to represent the core topics tested on the USMLE Step 1 and other standardized examinations. This text is not intended to replace comprehensive textbooks, course materials, or lectures. It is intended to be used as a valuable supplemental tool during your studies on microbiology and immunology whether it is for the USMLE Step 1 or classes. This book can be used as a tool to quiz both yourself and classmates on topics covered in recent lectures or clinical case discussions. A bookmark is included so that you can easily cover up the answers as you work through each chapter. The compact nature of the book is conducive to studying on the go, especially during any downtime you have during your busy day. We highly encourage you to use this book early and often as we believe repetition spread over a longer time frame results in better retention of knowledge. Last, we have provided a vast array of mnemonics within this text. These mnemonics include commonly known ones within the medical community as well as original ones created by ourselves during our own experiences studying for the USMLE Step 1. We hope you pick and choose which ones will best assist your studying. No matter how you choose to study, we hope this resource becomes helpful in your preparation for the USMLE Step 1. We wish you the best of luck studying!

Eric M. Chen
Joseph J. Chen

SECTION I

Basic Bacteriology

CHAPTER 1

General Principles (Structure, Genetics, Growth)

BACTERIAL STRUCTURES

What are the three major components of the bacterial envelope?	1. Capsule 2. Cell wall 3. Cell membrane
What macromolecule are bacterial capsules?	Polysaccharides (macromolecules made of sugar monomers)
What are the two notable examples of bacterial capsules made from a macromolecule other than polysaccharides?	1. The capsule of *Bacillus anthracis* is made from D-glutamic acid polypeptide. 2. The capsule of *Yersinia pestis* is made from amino acids.
What are the two functions of a bacterial capsule?	1. Capsules are virulence factors that serve to protect bacteria from phagocytosis by macrophages and neutrophils. 2. They also aid bacteria in attaching to host surfaces.
What test allows identification of a capsule in bacteria?	The Quellung test utilizes anti-capsular antibodies that bind and induce capsular swelling, which can then be visualized by light microscopy. It was used in the past for the detection of *Streptococcus pneumoniae*.
Why are capsules an important target for medical therapy?	Capsules contain polysaccharides that can be used for the development of vaccines such as the vaccine against *S. pneumoniae* and *Haemophilus influenzae* type B.

What macromolecule are bacterial cell walls made from?

The peptidoglycan murein, which is a polymer consisting of sugars and amino acids.

What is the major function of the cell wall?

The cell wall is a rigid structure that protects bacteria against mechanical forces such as osmotic gradients.

What is Gram staining?

Gram staining is a procedure by which bacteria can be classified by the ability of the cell wall to absorb a crystal violet dye, followed by a red safranin counter stain.

What color are gram-positive bacteria?

Gram-positive bacteria appear blue because they effectively absorb the crystal violet stain.

What color are gram-negative bacteria?

Gram-negative bacteria appear pink because they do not retain the crystal violet dye and take up the red safranin counter stain.

How do the peptidoglycan layers of gram-positive bacteria differ from those of gram-negative bacteria?

Gram-positive bacteria have thicker peptidoglycan cell walls (up to 90% of dry weight), whereas gram-negative bacteria have thinner peptidoglycan cell walls (about 10% of dry weight) with a periplasmic space.

What important enzyme is found in the periplasmic space of gram-negative bacteria?

β-Lactamase, an enzyme produced by bacteria that provide resistance to β-Lactam antibiotics such as penicillins and cephalosporins.

Pharmacology correlate: How do penicillins and cephalosporins work?

They bind to transpeptidase enzymes (also called penicillin-binding proteins) and prevent the cross-linking of sugar chains in the peptidoglycan murein (i.e., prevent synthesis of bacteria cell wall).

Which type of Gram-staining bacteria has teichoic and lipoteichoic acid? Which type has lipopolysaccharide (LPS)?

Teichoic and lipoteichoic acid—gram-positive bacteria. LPS (also known as endotoxin)—gram-negative bacteria

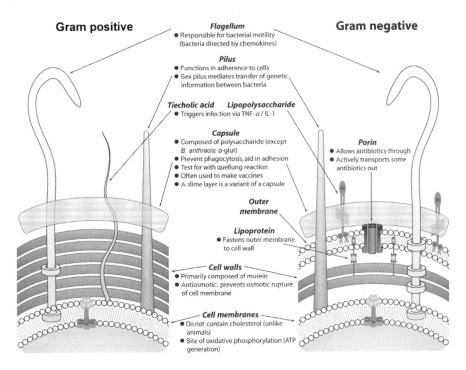

Gram positive

Gram negative

Flagellum
- Responsible for bacterial motility (bacteria directed by chemokines)

Pilus
- Functions in adherence to cells
- Sex pilus mediates transfer of genetic information between bacteria

Tiecholic acid   Lipopolysaccharide
- Triggers infection via TNF-α / IL-1

Capsule
- Composed of polysaccharide (except B. anthracis: D-glut)
- Prevent phagocytosis, aid in adhesion
- Test for with quellung reaction
- Often used to make vaccines
- A slime layer is a variant of a capsule

Porin
- Allows antibiotics through
- Actively transports some antibiotics out

Outer membrane

Lipoprotein
- Fastens outer membrane to cell wall

Cell walls
- Primarily composed of murein
- Antiosmotic: prevents osmotic rupture of cell membrane

Cell membranes
- Do not contain cholesterol (unlike animals)
- Site of oxidative phosphorylation (ATP generation)

Figure 1.1   Bacterial cell walls.

What are some of the pathologic effects of teichoic acid and LPS?	Both induce cytokines (e.g., tumor necrosis factor-α [TNF-α] and inter-leukin-1[IL-1]), which activate the inflammatory, complementary, and coagulation pathways, leading to septic shock (sepsis, fever, tachycardia, hypotension, and organ failure) and disseminated intravascular coagulation (DIC).
What are the three components of LPS?	1. Outer polysaccharide or O-antigen (the major surface antigen) 2. Middle core polysaccharide 3. Inner lipid A (phospholipid that causes the toxic effect)
What is the only gram-positive organism that has endotoxin?	*Listeria monocytogenes*
How do the cell walls of *Mycobacteria* species differ from those of gram-positive and gram-negative organisms?	*Mycobacteria* cell walls contain mycolic acids that do not Gram stain. Instead, they stain with carbolfuchsin (a component of Ziehl-Neelsen stain) and are called *acid-fast*.

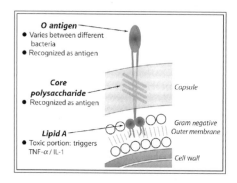

Figure 1.2   Lipopolysaccharide.

There are several bacteria that do not Gram stain. For each bacterium, name the alternate staining method:

Treponema	Dark-field microscopy and fluorescent antibody staining
Borrelia (relapsing fever)	Giemsa stain or dark-field microscopy
Legionella	Silver stain
Mycobacteria	Ziehl-Neelsen (acid-fast) stain
Rickettsia	Giemsa stain
Chlamydia	Giemsa, fluorescent antibody, and iodide staining

What bacteria lack a cell wall?   *Mycoplasma* species

How do bacterial cell membranes differ from mammalian cell membranes?   Bacterial cell membranes lack sterols (e.g., cholesterol) except for *Mycoplasma* species.

Since bacteria lack organelles such as mitochondria, where is the electron transport chain located?   Bacterial cell membrane

Bacteria use flagella to generate motion. What stimulus drives the direction of motion of flagellated bacteria?   Bacterial motion is dictated by chemical gradients (chemotaxis).

Name two bacteria with a single polar flagellum:
1. *Vibrio cholerae*
2. *Campylobacter jejuni*

What two bacteria have multiple flagella?
1. *Escherichia coli*
2. *Proteus mirabilis*

What are the two types of pili and what are their functions?	1. Common pili (fimbria) mediate bacterial adhesion. 2. Sex pili allow for exchange of genetic material.
What macromolecule is Glycocalyx, which allows bacteria to adhere to surfaces such as catheters, is made of?	Polysaccharides. Note that when the gycocalyx is tightly associated with the cell wall, it is known as a capsule; when it is loosely associated with the cell wall, it is known as a slime layer.
Name some pathogenic bacteria that utilize a slime layer glycocalyx for infection:	*Streptococcus mutans* (surfaces of teeth), *Streptococcus sanguis* (heart valves), *Staphylococcus epidermidis* (catheters)
What metabolically inactive structure formed by certain bacteria is resistant to environmental stresses?	Spore
What advantage does spore formation offer bacteria?	To ensure survival in a harsh environment. They are highly resistant to heat, chemicals, and radiation, making sterilization of medical equipment difficult (requiring use of autoclave).
What are the contents of an endospore?	Bacterial DNA with sparse cytoplasm, cell membrane, and peptidoglycan, encased in a thick, keratin-like coat
What two chemical features of spores allow for resistance to environmental stresses?	1. A keratin-like coat 2. Dipicolinic acid, found in the core of the endospore that helps in heat resistance
What are the two important spore-forming gram-positive rods?	1. *Bacillus* 2. *Clostridium* **Mnemonic:** Spores survive since **BC.**
Why are antibiotics not effective against spores?	Antibiotics cannot penetrate the spore coat and because of lack of metabolic activity, the antibiotics cannot act to inhibit the metabolic pathways of bacteria.
What is a fomite?	An inanimate object that can harbor and spread infections (e.g., blankets with smallpox or hospital bed rails with methicillin-resistant *Staphylococcus aureus* [MRSA]).

BACTERIAL GROWTH

What are the four phases of
bacterial growth?

1. Lag phase
2. Logarithmic phase (log)
3. Stationary phase
4. Death phase

During what phase do bacteria have
the highest metabolic activity but without cell division?

Lag phase

During what phase is growth the
fastest?

Log phase

During what phase do b-lactam drugs
act?

Log phases, inhibit synthesis of cell
walls

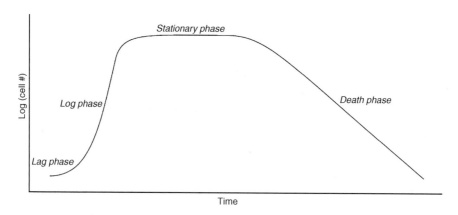

Phase	Description
Lag	Occurs when bacteria are transferred to new environment. Variable length. Bacteria may increase in size/mass, but division rate does not exceed death rate.
Log	Rapid cell division and exponential growth. (division rate > death rate)
Stationary	Aspect of environment no longer able to serve requirements of exponential growth (eg, depleting nutrient supply). Physiological adaptation of bacteria to survive through periods of declining resources. (division rate = death rate)
Death	Depletion of nutrients and buildup of toxic waste products lead to widespread death of bacteria. (division rate < death rate)

Figure 1.3   Bacterial growth curve.

In what phase does bacterial growth equal that of bacterial death?	Stationary phase
During what phase do spores form?	Stationary phase
During what phase have nutrient sources been exhausted?	Death phase
How are bacteria groups separated according to their oxygen requirements?	Obligate aerobes require oxygen for metabolism (e.g., *Pseudomonas*); facultative anaerobes can use aerobic or anaerobic metabolism (e.g., *Listeria*, *Enterobacteriaceae*); microaerophilic bacteria require low oxygen tension (e.g., *Campylobacter*); aerotolerant anaerobes can grow with or without oxygen, but only use anaerobic metabolism (*Enterococcus faecalis*); and obligate anaerobes cannot survive in oxygen (e.g., *Clostridium*).
What are some of the obligate aerobe bacteria?	Gram positive: *Nocardia*, *Bacillus* Gram negative: *Neisseria*, *Pseudomonas*, *Bordetella*, *Legionella*, *Brucella* Acid-fast: *Mycobacterium*, *Nocardia* (weakly acid-fast)
What are some of the obligate anaerobic bacteria?	Gram positive: *Clostridium*, *Actinomyces* Gram negative: *Bacteroides*
Why do obligate aerobes require oxygen?	Obligate aerobes require oxygen because their metabolism requires oxygen as the final electron acceptor. They use glycolysis, the tricarboxylic acid (TCA) cycle, and the electron transport chain.
How are facultative anaerobes different from obligate aerobes?	Facultative anaerobes are aerobic bacteria that have catalase and superoxide dismutase, so they can use oxygen as obligate aerobes. However, they can also grow in the absence of oxygen by using fermentation for energy.
How do microaerophilic bacteria tolerate low levels of oxygen?	They have superoxide dismutase, but no catalase.

Why are obligate anaerobes unable to grow in the presence of oxygen?	Because they do not have enzymes such as superoxide dismutase, catalase, or peroxidase to protect them from free O_2 radicals.
What are obligate intracellular organisms?	Organisms that can only survive within host cells (e.g., *Chlamydia* and *Rickettsia*) **Mnemonic: R**ob **C**ells of **ATP** (*Rickettsia*, *Chlamydia*)
How do obligate intracellular organisms generate ATP?	They cannot produce their own ATP, so they utilize the ATP of a host cell. Therefore, they can only survive within the host cell.
What are facultative intracellular organisms?	Organisms that can survive both intracellularly and extracellularly

BACTERIAL GENETICS

By what process do bacteria multiply?	Binary fission
Are bacteria haploid or diploid?	Haploid
Name two types of DNA forms found in bacteria:	1. Chromosomal DNA 2. Plasmid DNA
Name the location of chromosomal DNA in bacteria:	Nucleoid
Describe the DNA structure of plasmids:	Double-stranded circular DNA
Name some genes carried on plasmids:	Antibiotic resistance genes, pili genes, and exotoxin genes
How are plasmids transferred between bacteria?	Conjugation and transformation
What are the size and subunits for bacterial and eukaryotic ribosomes?	Bacterial: 70S with 50S and 30S subunits Eukaryotic: 80S with 60S and 40S subunits **Mnemonic:** Bacteria have three odd numbers in a row 3, 5, 7. Eukaryotes have three even numbers in a row 4, 6, 8.

Name four ways in which bacteria are able to acquire new genetic information:	1. Transformation 2. Transduction 3. Conjugation 4. Transposon insertion
How do bacteria acquire genetic information via transformation?	Bacteria take up DNA from the environment (e.g., living bacteria take up DNA from lysed bacteria).
What mediates the transfer of genetic material in transduction?	Bacteriophages (phages)
How do bacteriophages normally reproduce?	Bacteriophages inject bacteria with their phage DNA. Under the direction of the phage DNA, new bacteriophages are produced and are released by bacterial lysis.
How do bacteriophages transfer bacterial genetic material via transduction?	Newly produced phages are packaged with bacterial genes that are transferred to the next infected bacteria.
What are the two types of phages?	1. Virulent phage 2. Temperate phage
Which type of phage causes near-immediate lysis of bacteria?	Virulent phage
Unlike virulent phages, temperate phages undergo a period of inactivity, in which the phage DNA incorporates into the bacterial chromosomal DNA. What is the name of the incorporated phage DNA?	Prophage
Name the two types of transduction and the type of phage responsible for each:	1. Generalized (virulent phage) 2. Specialized (temperate phage)
What part of the bacterial chromosome is transferred in generalized transduction?	Any part of the bacterial genome
What part of the bacterial chromosome is transferred in specialized transduction?	The segment of the bacterial genome adjacent to the prophage of a temperate bacteriophage
Name some bacterial toxins acquired through specialized transduction:	Diphtheria toxin, botulinum toxin, cholera toxin, shiga-like toxin, and erythrogenic toxin

The sex pilus is the structure that allows for exchange of genetic material by conjugation. What types of DNA can be exchanged by conjugation?

Both chromosomal and plasmid

What plasmid encodes the proteins needed to form the sex pilus?

The F plasmid (F = fertility factor)

What is the term given when the F plasmid incorporates into the bacterial chromosomal DNA?

Hfr (high-frequency recombination)

Transposons are mobile segments of DNA that can insert into bacterial chromosomes and plasmids. Why are transposons medically relevant?

Transposons aid in the spread of antibiotic resistance.

Name a notable example of transposon-mediated drug resistance:

The *van*A transposon has given rise to vancomycin-resistant enterococci (VRE) and vancomycin-resistant *S. aureus* (VRSA).

What two bacteria undergo programmed rearrangement of surface antigens (antigenic variation) to avoid the host immune system?

1. *Neisseria gonorrhoeae*
2. *Borrelia recurrentis*

CHAPTER 2

Classification and Characteristics of Medically Important Bacteria and Normal Flora

What are the basic shape classifications of bacteria?	Cocci (spheres), bacilli (rods), and spirochetes (spirals)
What are the different pattern arrangements of cocci and common examples of each?	Diplococci (*Neisseria*), chains (streptococci), clusters (staphylococci)
What are the two main gram-positive cocci bacteria? What test differentiates them?	1. *Streptococcus*: catalase negative 2. *Staphylococcus*: catalase positive **Mnemonic: Cat**-in-**A-Staff** (*Staphylococcus aureus*)
What other bacteria are catalase positive?	Obligate aerobes (e.g., *Pseudomonas*), facultative anaerobes (e.g., *Listeria, Enterobacteriaceae*)
Name the clinically relevant *Staphylococcus* species. What two tests can be used to identify each one?	*Staphylococcus aureus*: coagulase positive 1. *Staphylococcus epidermidis*: coagulase negative, novobiocin sensitive 2. *Staphylococcus saprophyticus*: coagulase negative, novobiocin resistant
Sheep blood agar is used to differentiate *Streptococcus* with α, β, and γ hemolysis. Describe these different types of hemolysis.	γ: No hemolysis, α: partial hemolysis (green color), β: complete hemolysis with central clearing due to hemolysin enzymes

Name some bacteria that display α, β, and γ hemolysis:

α Hemolysis: *Streptococcus pneumoniae, Streptococcus viridans,* and some enterococci

β Hemolysis: *Streptococcus pyogenes, Streptococcus agalactiae, S. aureus, Listeria monocytogenes*

γ Hemolysis: some enterococci

Lancefield group antigens are carbohydrates present in the cell walls of *Streptococcus* species and serve as a means of classification. Name the bacteria associated with the following Lancefield antigens:

Group A

S. pyogenes

Group B

S. agalactiae

Group D

Streptococcus bovis and enterococci (*Enterococcus faecalis* and *Enterococcus faecium*). Note that *Enterococcus* was split from the *Streptococcus* genus in the late 1980s and is now its own genus.

Which Group D bacteria, *Streptococcus* or *Enterococcus,* can grow in hypertonic (6.5%) saline? Which cannot?

Enterococci can grow in hypertonic saline and *S. bovis* cannot.

What tests can differentiate *S. pneumoniae* from *S. viridans*?

Streptococcus pneumoniae: optochin (detergent-like compound) sensitive, bile soluble, and Quellung test positive
Streptococcus viridans: optochin resistant, not bile soluble, and Quellung negative

Mnemonic: optochin disk is also called the **P** disk = P*neumococcus*

What test can differentiate *S. pyogenes* and *S. agalactiae*?

Bacitracin (an antibiotic) sensitivity. *Streptococcus pyogenes* is bacitracin sensitive and *S. agalactiae* is bacitracin resistant.

Mnemonic: bacitracin disk is also called the **A** disk = group **A** Strep (*S. pyogenes*)

What are the clinically relevant gram-positive bacilli? Which one(s) form spores? Which one(s) are obligate aerobes and which one(s) are anaerobes?

Corynebacterium, Listeria, Bacillus, and *Clostridium. Bacillus* and *Clostridium* form spores. *Bacillus* is an obligate aerobe while *Clostridium* is an obligate anaerobe.

Which gram-positive bacillus has metachromatic granules? What are the granules composed of?

Corynebacterium diphtheriae. The granules are composed of phosphate inclusions.

Name two filamentous fungi-like gram-positive bacteria. Which one is an obligate aerobe and which one is an obligate anaerobe?

1. *Nocardia*: obligate aerobe, weakly acid fast
2. *Actinomyces*: obligate anaerobe

What are the clinically relevant gram-negative cocci bacteria?

Neisseria meningitidis, Neisseria gonorrhoeae, Moraxella catarrhalis, and *Acinetobacter baumannii*

Name two important distinctions between *N. meningitidis* and *N. gonorrhoeae*:

1. *Neisseria meningitidis* has a capsule (and therefore a vaccine) and reduces maltose.
2. *Neisseria gonorrhoeae* does not have a capsule (or a vaccine) and cannot reduce maltose.

Mnemonic: *N. meningitidis* = **M**altose reducer

What are some clinically relevant gram-negative bacilli bacteria?

Think of groups: enterics (*Escherichia, Vibrio, Helicobacter, Campylobacter, Salmonella, Shigella*), respiratory pathogens (*Bordetella, Legionella, Haemophilus, Klebsiella, Pseudomonas*), and zoonotics (*Francisella, Brucella, Bartonella, Yersinia, Pasteurella*)

Mnemonics: Enterics are **V**ery **H**ellish **C**ompany in the **S**tomach and **S**tool (*E*scherichia, *V*ibrio, *H*elicobacter, *C*ampylobacter, *S*almonella, *S*higella)

Keep **B**reathing a **L**ittle **H**arder **P**lease (*K*lebsiella, *B*ordetella, *L*egionella, *H*aemophilus, *P*seudomonas)

Find **Bru**tal **Ba**cteria on **Y**our **P**ets (*Fra*cisella, *Bru*cella, *Ba*rtonella *Y*ersinia, *P*asteurella)

What gram-negative bacilli belong to Enterobacteriaceae family?

Escherichia, Proteus, Serratia, Enterobacter, Klebsiella, Shigella, Salmonella, Yersinia

Mnemonic: Enterobacteriaceae are **PESSKY** **S**trains of bacteria (*E*nterobacter, *P*roteus, *E*scherichia, *S*hig*ella*, *S*almon*ella*, *K*lebsi*ella*, *Y*ersinia, *S*erratia) three ELLAs in a row

What three antigens are used for serotyping of Enterobacteriaceae?

1. O antigen (cell wall component of endotoxin)
2. H antigen (flagella antigen, only on motile species)
3. K antigen (capsule antigen, also used for virulence of *Salmonella typhi*)

What features define the Enterobacteriaceae?

Gram-negative rods, *glucose fermenting* therefore *oxidase negative* (i.e., lack cytochrome c involved in electron transport chain of oxidation), *facultative anaerobes* therefore catalase positive, and *nitrite positive* (e.g., reduce nitrate to nitrite in metabolic processes)

What features define Pseudomonas?

Gram-negative rods, *nonglucose fermenting*, *oxidase positive* (i.e., have cytochrome c since necessary to oxidize glucose), *obligate aerobes* therefore also catalase positive, and *nitrite negative*

What bacteria are urease positive? What does urease do?

Helicobacter pylori, Proteus, Ureaplasma, Nocardia, and some strains of *Pseudomonas* and *Kiebsiella*. Urease degrades urea into ammonia and carbon dioxide.

Mnemonic: *Corynebacterium urealyticum*, H. *Pylori, Ureaplasma, Nocardia, Kiebsiella* (some), *Proteus, Pseudomonas* (some) (**CHUNKy PP**)

What are the common spirochetes?

Treponema, Borrelia, and *Leptospira*

What shape are spirochetes?

Spiral-shaped rods

Are spirochetes mobile?

Yes, movement of internal filaments propels these bacteria.

What type of microscopy is used to visualize spirochetes?

Typically dark-field microscopy because spirochetes do not stain well with traditional stains. However, silver or fluorescence stain can also be used.

NORMAL BACTERIAL FLORA

What is a *carrier state*?

A person with an asymptomatic infection or who has recovered from an infection but continues to carry the organism and may shed it.

What occurs in *colonization* **of an individual?**

The acquisition and replication of a new organism not part of the normal flora that may cause an infection or be eliminated by host defenses. Patients do not present with symptoms.

What are the benefits of normal flora?

Normal flora occupies attachment sites on skin and mucosa and thus prevents colonization by pathogenic bacteria. They also supply nutrients by producing several B vitamins and vitamin K.

What is the predominant organism of the skin and when can it be pathogenic?

Staphylococcus epidermidis. It can be pathogenic when it implants on devices such as artificial heart valves and prosthetic joints.

What yeast, which is a normal flora of the skin, can cause systemic infections in those with reduced cell-mediated immunity?

Candida species. Remember to think causes of reduced immunity such as diabetes, cancers, human immunodeficiency virus (HIV), etc.

What common skin anaerobe plays a role in the pathogenesis of acne?

Propionibacterium acnes

What common bacterial group, which is normally found in the oral cavity, is the leading cause of subacute bacterial endocarditis, especially in patients with preexisting valvular disease?

Streptococcus viridans

What do the anaerobic bacteria of the gastrointestinal (GI) tract, such as *Clostridium* and *Bacteroides*, commonly cause if aspirated?

Lung abscesses

Where in the body does *S. aureus* commonly colonize?

The nose—specifically the anterior nares

What are some normal flora of the intestinal tract that are pathogenic?

Escherichia coli (urinary tract infections [UTIs], diarrhea, neonatal meningitis, hemolytic-uremic syndrome), *Bacteroides fragilis* (peritonitis), *Enterococcus faecalis* (UTIs, endocarditis), *Pseudomonas aeruginosa* (various infections particularly hospitalized patients)

When a patient is treated with clindamycin or other broad-spectrum antibiotics, what organism commonly overgrows the colon, sometimes leading to pseudomembranous colitis?

Clostridium difficile. Treat with either oral vancomycin or metronidazole.

What is the predominant bacterial species in normal vaginal flora of adult women? What common fungus's overgrowth is suppressed by this normal flora?

Lactobacillus species prevent overgrowth by *Candida albicans*.

What is the predominant organism of the urethra?

Staphylococcus epidermidis

CHAPTER 3

Pathogenesis and Host Defense

What are the two broad systems of defense against pathogens in the human body?

1. Innate or nonspecific immunity
2. Adaptive or specific immunity (for more detail refer to Chapters 37, 39, and 40)

Name the major constituents of innate immunity:

Physical barriers (skin and mucous membranes), soluble factors (complement and cytokines), physiologic factors (temperature, pH), and cellular defenses (natural killer [NK] cells and neutrophils)

Apart from being a physical barrier, what are the other antimicrobial properties of the skin?

Mildly acidic (pH 5–6), normal body temperature, dry, endogenous antimicrobial peptides, and normal skin flora (compete with pathogens)

Name some antimicrobial substances found in mucus:

Lysozyme, immunoglobulin A (IgA) antibodies, and iron-binding proteins

What is the target of lysozyme?

Peptidoglycan structure of gram-positive cell walls

What is the function of the secretory component of IgA?

Protection from proteolysis

What are some components of respiratory defenses?

Filtration of particles in the upper airways (nose hairs and mucus), mucociliary apparatus, cough reflex, mucus, and alveolar macrophages

Name some bacteria that specifically target the mucociliary apparatus:

Bordetella pertussis, Haemophilus influenzae, Pseudomonas aeruginosa, Mycoplasma pneumoniae

What are some nonimmunological components of intestinal defense?

Acid in stomach, pancreatic enzymes, bile, Paneth cells (secrete defensins and lysozymes), and peristalsis

What is the major mechanism of defense of the vagina?

Acidic environment created by vaginal flora

What kind of immune response is elicited by capsular polysaccharide?

B cells generate T-cell–independent antibodies to aid macrophages in phagocytosis (opsonization).

Why does splenectomy predispose to more severe infections with encapsulated organisms?

The spleen is a lymphoid organ containing B cells and macrophages needed to effectively clear encapsulated organisms. Severe fulminant infections with *Streptococcus pneumoniae*, *Neisseria*, and *Haemophilus* are more common following splenectomy.

What diseases are potentially treated with splenectomy?

Hereditary spherocytosis, idiopathic thrombocytopenic purpura, and trauma

What disease is associated with autosplenectomy?

Sickle cell anemia

What is the role of complement in innate immunity?

Opsonization/phagocytosis, cytolysis, and chemotaxis

Macrophages release various cytokines in innate immunity. Name the function of the following cytokines:

  Tumor necrosis factor-α (TNF-α)

  Induces the inflammatory response

  Interleukin-1 (IL-1)

  Induces fever, which enhances the immune response

  Interleukin-6 (IL-6)

  Induces the acute-phase response

  Interleukin-8 (IL-8)

  Chemotactic factor neutrophils

  Interlukin-12 (IL-12)

  Activates NK and Th1 cells

The acute-phase response represents a group of proteins released from the liver as part of innate immunity. Name the function of the following acute-phase proteins:

  C-reactive protein

  Clears necrotic debris by binding to dead cells and activating the classical complement pathway

  Haptoglobin

  Conserves body iron by binding hemoglobin

  Fibrinogen

  Limits spread of bacteria

What immune cells are involved in innate immunity?

NK cells, neutrophils, macrophages

What group of receptors allows neutrophils and macrophages to recognize conserved bacterial structures such as lipopolysaccharide (LPS)?

Toll-like receptors (pattern-recognition receptors)

By what mechanism do neutrophils and monocytes engulf bacteria and kill them?

Oxygen-dependent (respiratory burst) and oxygen-independent (muramidase, lactoferrin, low pH, lysozyme)

What enzyme produces superoxide ($O_2 \bullet^-$) from oxygen (O_2)?

Nicotinamide adenine dinucleotide phosphate (NADPH) oxidase in the neutrophil cell membrane

What enzyme converts superoxide ($O_2 \bullet^-$) to peroxide (H_2O_2)?

Superoxide dismutase

What enzyme degrades peroxide (H_2O_2) into H_2O and oxygen, and thereby protects bacteria?

Catalase

What enzyme forms hypochlorite (HOCL$\bullet^-$) from peroxide (H_2O_2) and chloride (Cl^-)?

Myeloperoxidase. Hypochlorite is 50 times more potent than peroxide at killing bacteria.

In addition to respiratory bursts, what other free radical-generating system is found in macrophages?

Inducible nitric oxide synthase (iNOS) produces nitric oxide (NO).

CHAPTER 4

Laboratory Diagnosis

For each bacteria, name the appropriate agar:

Bordetella pertussis	Bordet-Gengou
Mycobacterium tuberculosis	Lowenstein-Jensen
Neisseria gonorrhoeae	Thayer-Martin
Corynebacterium diphtheriae	Tellurite and Loeffler

For each agar, name the appropriate bacteria:

Egg yolk	*Clostridium perfringens*
Charcoal yeast with iron and cysteine	*Legionella pneumophila*
Chocolate agar with factors V and X	*Haemophilus influenzae*
MacConkey and eosin-methylene blue (EMB)	Gram-negative lactose fermenters (*Escherichia coli*, *Enterobacter*, *Klebsiella*, *Serratia*, *Vibrio*), pink on MacConkey and green on EMB. Non–lactose-fermenting gram-negative rods have clear, nonpink colonies on MacConkey. **Mnemonic: SEEK V**erification (*Serratia*, *E. coli*, *Enterobacter*, *Klebsiella*, *Vibrio*)

Which bacteria produce a black pigment on Bile-Esculin Agar?

Group D streptococci and enterococci

What does the Quellung test detect?

Capsule. Quellung is the German word for "swelling."

Name some bacteria that are Quellung positive:

Cryptococcus (not bacteria), *Pseudomonas*, *Neisseria meningitidis*, *H. influenzae*, *Klebsiella*, and *Streptococcus pneumoniae* **Mnemonic: C**apsules **P**rotect **N**aughty **H**uman **K**illing **S**trains of bacteria

What other tests are used to determine the presence of a capsule? How do the tests work?

Latex agglutination. Latex beads complexed to antibodies precipitate when they bind the capsular antigen of interest. This test is usually used to aid in diagnosis of bacterial meningitis. Wet mount with India ink also can be used to identify *Cryptococcus* capsule.

What bacteria is identified by the Elek test? How does the Elek test work?

Corynebacterium diphtheriae. Antitoxin (antibody to diphtheria toxin)-coated strips are placed onto agar with *C. diphtheriae* inoculated at right angles to the antitoxin strips. If toxigenic *C. diphtheriae* is present, toxin-antitoxin complexes precipitate.

How does ELISA (enzyme-linked immunosorbent assay) work?

An enzyme linked to either a bacterial antigen or antibody reacts in direct proportion to the amount of antigen-antibody complexes formed.

Describe direct and indirect immunofluorescence.

Direct immunofluorescence detects specific *bacterial antigens* by using antibodies conjugated with fluorescent dyes to directly bind the bacterial antigen, which then causes fluorescence under ultraviolet (UV) light.

Indirect immunofluorescence detects *serum antibodies* by using known antigens to bind the antibodies, which can then be detected under UV light by antihuman IgG antibodies conjugated with fluorescent dyes.

Name two types of bacteria that are identified by immunofluorescence:

1. *Chlamydia*
2. Spirochetes

How does polymerase chain reaction (PCR) work?

PCR amplifies bacterial DNA using bacterial-specific primers, free DNA bases, and DNA polymerase, allowing for identification of bacteria.

What bacterial species causes IgM cold autoimmune antibodies?

Mycoplasma pneumoniae

What are the two nonspecific tests (to detect nonspecific antibodies) for syphilis?

1. VDRL (Venereal Disease Research Laboratory)
2. RPR (rapid plasma reagin)

What disease states may cause a false-positive result with a nonspecific syphilis test?

Hepatitis B, infectious mononucleosis, leprosy, and autoimmune diseases such as systemic lupus erythematosus

What are the two specific tests (to detect disease-specific antibodies) for syphilis?

1. FTA-ABS (fluorescent treponemal antibody-absorbed test)
2. MHA-TP (microhemagglutination-*Treponema pallidum*)

CHAPTER 5

Antimicrobial Drugs and Vaccines

INHIBITORS OF CELL WALL & CELL MEMBRANE

Name the major categories of β-lactam antibiotics:	Penicillins, cephalosporins, mono-bactams, and carbapenems
What is the mechanism of action of all β-lactam antibiotics?	They bind to and permanently inactivate transpeptidases (sometimes known as penicillin-binding proteins), which are involved in bacterial cell wall synthesis.
What is the difference between penicillins G and V? What is the most common adverse effect of penicillin?	Penicillin G is given intravenously and penicillin V is resistant to gastric acid, allowing it to be given orally. Hypersensitivity reactions ($< 1\%–8\%$) are the most common adverse effect.
Which bacteria are potentially susceptible to penicillin G?	Gram positives (with exceptions such as *Staphylococcus aureus*), *Neisseria*, spirochetes, and most anaerobes
	Mnemonic: penicillin G treatment **SPAN**s (**S**pirochetes, gram **p**ositives, **A**naerobes, *Neisseria*)
How does probenecid increase the half-life of penicillin G?	It blocks active renal secretion of penicillin.
Which penicillins are the semisynthetic (anti-*Staph*) penicillins that are potentially more resistant to β-lactamases?	Methicillin, nafcillin, oxacillin, cloxacillin, and dicloxacillin

What is the Jarisch-Herxheimer phenomenon?

Acute worsening of symptoms (fever, headache, muscle pains) soon after penicillin G treatment due to released pyrogens from killed organisms, especially with treatment of syphilis

Which penicillin class can be used to treat *Pseudomonas aeruginosa*?

Carbenicillin and ticarcillin (the carboxypenicillins), and piperacillin, mezlocillin, and azlocillin (the ureidopenicillins)

Do β-lactamase inhibitors such as clavulanic acid or tazobactam improve activity of β-lactams against β-lactam–resistant *P. aeruginosa*?

No, β-lactamase inhibitors do not generally improve the activity of β-lactams against *Pseudomonas*. Resistance is generally by mechanisms other than β-lactamases.

Which organisms can be treated by use of Ampicillin or amoxicillin?

Haemophilus influenzae, Escherichia coli, Listeria monocytogenes, Proteus mirabilis, Salmonella, Borrelia burgdorferi, and enterococci. Strains resistant to ampicillin are becoming more common.

Mnemonic: Ampicillin/amoxicillin **HELPS** kill enterococci (*H. influenzae, E. coli, Listeria, Proteus,* and *Salmonella*)

What is the standard treatment of meningitis caused by *L. monocytogenes*?

Ampicillin and gentamicin

What are the potential problems with cephalosporins that contain *N*-methylthiotetrazole side chains?

Disulfiram-like reaction causing hypotension, nausea, and vomiting when ingested with ethanol and prolonged prothrombin time because of interference with vitamin K activity leading to increased risk of bleeds

Which cephalosporin antibiotics have the best coverage against *P. aeruginosa*?

Cefepime (fourth generation) and ceftazidime (third generation)

Which cephalosporin antibiotics are often used for the treatment of community-acquired meningitis? Why?

Ceftriaxone (third generation) and cefotaxime (third generation) because they can readily cross the blood-brain barrier and cover most strains of *Streptococcus pneumoniae* and *Neisseria meningitidis* (most common causes of adult community-acquired meningitis)

Which cephalosporins are commonly used as prophylaxis for gastrointestinal (GI) surgery? Why?

Cefoxitin (second generation) and cefotetan (second generation) because they have activity against anaerobes and enteric gram-negative rods

Why are penicillins and cephalosporins ineffective against *Mycoplasma pneumoniae*?

Mycoplasma does not have cell walls.

Which β-lactam antibiotic is safe for the treatment of gram-negative organisms such as *Pseudomonas* in patients with penicillin allergies?

Aztreonam (monobactams)

What are the only types of bacteria susceptible to aztreonam?

Aerobic gram-negative bacteria

Why is imipenem, which has the broadest coverage of all the β-lactam drugs, always given with cilastatin?

Cilastatin is a dehydropeptidase inhibitor that inhibits metabolism of imipenem in the kidneys. This prevents nephrotoxicity and increases the urine concentration of intact imipenem, allowing for therapy of urinary tract infections.

What is the chief concern of having high plasma levels of imipenem?

Central nervous system (CNS) toxicity/ seizures

What are the advantages of meropenem over imipenem?

Meropenem does not need to be administered with cilastatin and causes fewer seizures.

How do bacteria become resistant to β-lactam drugs?

Production of β-lactamases, mutations in transpeptidases (penicillin-binding proteins), or altered porins

Which drug is the treatment of choice for methicillin-resistant *S. aureus* (MRSA) and what are its major side effects?

Vancomycin. Nephrotoxicity, ototoxicity, thrombophlebitis, diffuse erythema due to histamine release, and DRESS syndrome.

Mnemonic: NOTE the side effects of vancomycin (**N**ephrotoxicity, **O**totoxicity, **T**hrombophlebitis, and diffuse **E**rythema)

How do certain gram-positive bacteria become resistant to vancomycin?

By mutation of the terminal D-alanine-D-alanine sequence in bacterial cell wall to which vancomycin binds. Vancomycin inhibits cell wall synthesis but it is not a β-lactam drug.

What is the mechanism of action of bacitracin? What preparation is used clinically?

Prevents dephosphorylation and thus regeneration of a phospholipid carrier needed for cell wall synthesis. Topical agent (too toxic for systemic use)

Cycloserine is a second-line agent for tuberculosis. What is the mechanism of action of cycloserine? What are its side effects?

Analog of D-alanine that prevents the formation of the D-alanyl-D-alanine dipeptide in cell wall synthesis. CNS toxicity: seizures, acute psychosis, and peripheral neuropathy

Mnemonic: PSYCHO-serine due to CNS side effects

What is the mechanism of action of fosfomycin which is used for UTIs?

Inhibits enolpyruvate transferase, preventing the formation of N-acetylmuramic (NAM) acid

What is the mechanism of action of daptomycin?

Disrupts cell membranes polarity by opening transmembrane channels

Why can't daptomycin be used to treat pneumonia?

Surfactant binds to daptomycin, inactivating it.

What are some side effects of daptomycin?

Myopathy and rhabodmyolysis (when used with statins) and CPK elevation.

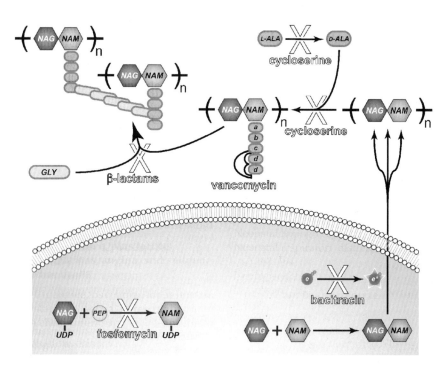

Figure 5.1   Bacterial cell wall synthesis.

INHIBITORS OF PROTEIN SYNTHESIS

Which antibiotics target the 30S and 50S ribosomal subunits respectively?

30S: aminoglycosides (neomycin, amikacin, tobramycin, gentamicin) and tetracyclines (minocycline, doxycycline)

50S: chloramphenicol, macrolides (erythromycin, azithromycin, clarithromycin), clindamycin, linezolid, streptogramins

What is the mechanism of action of aminoglycosides?

They inhibit translation by disrupting the formation of ribosomal initiation complex and cause misreading of the mRNA.

Why are aminoglycosides ineffective against anaerobic bacteria?

They require oxygen for uptake into the bacterium.

What is the benefit and mechanism of giving β-lactam antibiotics with aminoglycosides?

β-Lactam antibiotics facilitate the entry of aminoglycosides into bacterial cells by damaging the cell wall.

Which aminoglycoside is often given orally before GI surgery because it is poorly absorbed and prevents organisms from reaching the peritoneal cavity?

Neomycin. It is effective against gram-negative enteric flora.

What are the common side effects of aminoglycosides?

Nephrotoxicity (6%–7%), ototoxicity (2%; more common with loop diuretics), birth defects (teratogen), and neuromuscular blockade via decreased acetylcholine (ACh) release. Contraindicated in patients with Graves disease.

Mnemonic: aminoglycosides **N**eed **O**xygen **T**o **W**ork = **N**ephrotoxicity, **O**totoxicity, **T**eratogen, **W**eakness

How do bacteria usually become resistant to aminoglycosides?

Enzymatically inactivate aminoglycosides by conjugation (most important mechanism because this can be transferred between bacteria by transposons or plasmids). Aminoglycoside resistance may also be due to ribosome alteration or decreased cell permeability to aminoglycosides.

What species of bacteria are generally susceptible to tetracyclines?

Chlamydia, Mycoplasma, Rickettsia, Borrelia burgdorferi, E. coli, Neisseria gonorrhoeae, Vibrio, streptococci, community-acquired methicillin-resistant *S. aureus, Legionella, Brucella , Propionibacterium acnes*

What are some important side effects of tetracyclines?

Photosensitivity, staining of teeth (avoid in children), liver dysfunction in pregnant women, esophageal irritation (ulceration), and vertigo

Tetracyclines are commonly used to treat which common dermatological condition in teenagers?

Acne vulgaris

Which tetracycline can be used in the treatment of SIADH (syndrome of inappropriate antidiuretic hormone)? Why?

Demeclocycline causes nephrogenic diabetes insipidus by blocking antidiuretic hormone (ADH) receptor in the renal collecting ducts.

What is unique about doxycycline in comparison with other tetracyclines in regard to the means of elimination?

Doxycycline is eliminated in the feces (70%–80%) and is not dependent on either the liver or kidneys. It is safe for a patient with liver and kidney dysfunction and dose adjustments are not necessary.

Why should tetracyclines be taken on an empty stomach?

They can be chelated and inactivated by calcium, magnesium, aluminum, iron, and other multivalent cations.

Do tetracyclines work synergistically with penicillins?

Unlike aminoglycosides, tetracyclines theoretically decrease the effect of penicillins.

What is the risk from taking expired tetracyclines?

May cause a Fanconi-like syndrome (proximal renal tubular dysfunction)

How do bacteria usually become resistant to tetracyclines?

Increased ability to *pump* tetracycline out of cell (efflux pumps), decreased uptake, and enzymatic inactivation.

What is the mechanism of action of chloramphenicol? For which conditions is it used?

It prevents peptide bond formation by binding the 50S subunit of rRNA. It is used for bacterial meningitis in penicillin-allergic patients and serious *Salmonella* infections in some parts of the world.

What are the two distinct side effects of chloramphenicol on bone marrow?

1. Dose-dependent bone marrow suppression
2. Dose-independent aplastic anemia

It also causes *gray baby* syndrome in neonates because they lack uridine diphosphate (UDP)-glucuronyl transferase.

What is the mechanism of action of macrolide (erythromycin, azithromycin, clarithromycin) antibiotics?

They bind to the 50S ribosomal subunit and prevent the translocation step in protein synthesis.

Mnemonic: Macro**lide** stops the s**lide**

Why are macrolides used for the treatment of community-acquired pneumonia?

They are effective in treating *M. pneumoniae, Chlamydia pneumoniae, S. pneumoniae,* and *Legionella pneumophilia;* so they effectively cover the most common causes of community-acquired pneumonia.

How do bacteria usually become resistant to macrolides?

It is because of methyltransferases that alter the drug-binding site on the 50S ribosome and increase active transport of the drug out of the cell.

What is the mechanism of action of clindamycin?

Blocks peptide bond formation at the 50S ribosomal subunit. It is bacteriostatic.

What is the major side effect of clindamycin?

Pseudomembranous colitis due to overgrowth of *Clostridium difficile.* Remember, clindamycin isn't the most common cause of pseudomembranous colitis because it's not used as much as cephalosporins or ampicillin.

What is the mechanism of action for linezolid?

Inhibits the formation of the initiation complex in bacterial translation

What important infections does linezolid treat?

Vancomycin-resistant *S. aureus* (VRSA), methicillin-resistant *S. aureus* (MRSA), and vancomycin-resistant enterococci (VRE)

INHIBITORS OF NUCLEIC ACID REPLICATION

What is the mechanism of action of fluoroquinolones (ciprofloxacin, norfloxacin)?

Inhibit DNA gyrase (topoisomerase II), leading to inhibition of DNA replication and breakdown of DNA. They are bactericidal.

What are common indications for fluoroquinolones?

Urinary tract infections (UTIs), sexually transmitted diseases (STDs) (*Chlamydia* and *N. gonorrhoeae*), diarrhea (enterotoxigenic *E. coli* [ETEC], *Shigella*, *Salmonella*, and *Campylobacter*), and pneumonia (*Mycoplasma*, *Legionella*)

How does resistance to fluoroquinolones develop?

Resistance develops by point mutations of the DNA gyrase enzyme.

Why are fluoroquinolones contraindicated in pregnant women and in children?

Interfere with cartilage formation. In elderly, associated with Achilles tendonitis/tendon rupture

INHIBITORS OF FOLIC ACID SYNTHESIS

Name two antibiotics that inhibit bacterial growth by acting as *p*-aminobenzoic acid (PABA) analogs:

1. Sulfonamides
2. Dapsone

Which enzyme in bacterial folate synthesis is inhibited by sulfonamides?

Dihydropteroate synthetase

Can bacteria obtain folic acid by diffusion or active transport?

No, bacteria must synthesize folic acid from PABA.

What is the main risk of giving sulfonamides during pregnancy?

Sulfonamides can displace bilirubin from plasma albumin-binding sites and induce kernicterus in the newborn.

What are some other side effects of sulfonamides?

Induce hemolysis in glucose-6-phosphate dehydrogenase (G6PD)-deficient patients, megaloblastic anemia, photosensitivity, and hypersensitivities

What is the mechanism of action of trimethoprim?

Inhibits bacterial dihydrofolate reductase

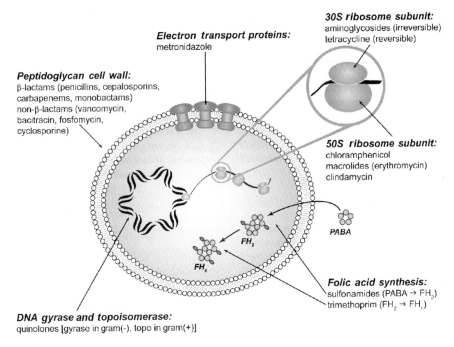

30S ribosome subunit:
aminoglycosides (irreversible)
tetracycline (reversible)

Electron transport proteins:
metronidazole

Peptidoglycan cell wall:
β-lactams (penicillins, cepalosporins,
carbapenems, monobactams)
non-β-lactams (vancomycin,
bacitracin, fosfomycin,
cyclosporine)

50S ribosome subunit:
chloramphenicol
macrolides (erythromycin)
clindamycin

FH_2

PABA

FH_4

Folic acid synthesis:
sulfonamides (PABA → FH_2)
trimethoprim (FH_2 → FH_4)

DNA gyrase and topoisomerase:
quinolones [gyrase in gram(-), topo in gram(+)]

Figure 5.2   Antibacterial targets.

What are important side effects of trimethoprim?

Adverse effects include megaloblastic anemia, leukopenia, and granulocytopenia. Alleviate these symptoms with supplemental folinic acid.

What is the drug of choice for treating simple recurrent UTIs?

Trimethoprim-sulfamethoxazole (TMP-SMX). Give ciprofloxacin if patient has sulfa allergy.

TREATMENT OF *MYCOBACTERIUM*

Which drugs are commonly used to treat *Mycobacterium tuberculosis* infection?

Ethambutol, rifampin, isoniazid (INH), and pyrazinamide (RIPE therapy)

What is the mechanism of action of ethambutol and what is its unique side effect?

Inhibits arabinosyl transferase, an enzyme necessary to make the mycobacterial cell wall. Also causes decreased visual acuity and color vision

What is the mechanism of action of rifampin?

Inhibits DNA-dependent RNA polymerase by binding to RNA polymerase and blocking elongation of RNA

What are common indications for rifampin?

Treatment of *M. tuberculosis* and prophylaxis for *N. meningitidis* or *H. influenzae*

Why shouldn't rifampin be used as monotherapy?

Resistance occurs rapidly when used as monotherapy. It can be used alone briefly for *N. meningitidis* or *H. influenzae* prophylaxis.

What are some common side effects of rifampin?

Induces P450 potentially leading to impaired efficacy of other drugs, GI symptoms, headache, fever, rash, red-orange urine.

What are the 4 R's of rifampin?

Red urine, **R**amps up P450 system, **R**esistance if given alone, **R**NA polymerase inhibitor

What is the mechanism of action for INH?

Although not proven, it is thought to inhibit mycolic acid synthesis

What are important side effects of INH?

Hepatotoxicity (avoid alcohol), peripheral neuropathy (vitamin B_6 depletion), sideroblastic anemia (vitamin B_6 depletion)

Name the three drugs commonly used in the treatment of leprosy:

1. Dapsone
2. Rifampin
3. Clofazimine

Which antibiotic is a PABA analog with a side-effect profile that includes hemolysis and methemoglobinemia?

Dapsone

Methemoglobinemia occurs when the ferrous (Fe^{2+}) form of iron in hemoglobin is oxidized to the ferric (Fe^{3+}) form and cannot bind O_2. What are the clinical manifestations of methemoglobinemia?

Dyspnea, headaches, dizziness, altered mental status with cyanosis of extremities, and darkened blood. Treat with methylene blue.

VACCINES

What is a live-attenuated vaccine?

Attenuated vaccine has microbe with selective deletions of genes involved in pathogenesis. Organisms replicate in the host, greatly increasing antigenic stimulation.

What are the advantages of live-attenuated vaccines?

A single inoculation may lead to lifelong immunity. Mucosal immunity possible with oral administration of some live-attenuated organisms. Increased potential for herd immunity compared with killed vaccines.

What are the disadvantages of live-attenuated vaccines?

Reversion to wild-type is a rare but serious complication, especially in immunocompromised patients. Contamination by live organisms or toxins is also a rare but serious consequence.

What is a killed vaccine?

Killed vaccines contain organisms inactivated by chemical or physical means.

What are the major advantages of killed vaccines?

They are significantly safer than attenuated vaccines in immunocompromised hosts.

What are the major disadvantages of killed vaccines?

Multiple doses must be given; immunity is not lifelong; and adjuvants are often required to further stimulate immune response to the antigens.

What is bacillus Calmette-Guérin (BCG) vaccine?

Live-attenuated *Mycobacterium bovis* vaccine often used in countries where tuberculosis is endemic. Shown effective for prevention of miliary and meningeal tuberculosis.

What type of vaccine is the *H. influenzae* vaccine?

It is a conjugated vaccine to diphtheria toxoid against the serotype B (the polysaccharide capsule in 95% of invasive strains).

Which polymer substance normally found in the organism's capsule in the polysaccharide antigen is used in the H. influenzae vaccine?

Polyribosylribitol phosphate (PRP)

What type of vaccine is the S. pneumoniae vaccine?

There are two types of vaccines available for S. pneumoniae. The first vaccine is composed of 23 polysaccharides purified from the capsules of the most important serotypes. This vaccine is indicated for at-risk adults (>65 years old, asplenic) and the antibody levels decrease to prevaccination levels after 10 years. The second vaccine is the 13-valent conjugate vaccine that is recommended for all infants and children.

In addition to the H. influenzae and S. pneumoniae vaccines, name two other bacterial vaccines consisting of capsular polysaccharides:

1. Neisseria meningitidis
2. Salmonella typhi

In what forms are the diphtheria and tetanus vaccines administered?

They are given as toxoids, a nontoxic derivative of a bacterial exotoxin that retains most of their antigenic properties.

Which two bacterial vaccines contain purified bacterial proteins?

1. Acellular pertussis
2. Anthrax vaccines

For the treatment and prevention of which bacterial diseases is passive immunity in the form of antitoxins used?

Tetanus, botulism, diphtheria

Why should tetanus antitoxin and tetanus toxoid be given at separate sites when administering as posttetanus exposure prophylaxis?

So that the antibodies in the antitoxin do not neutralize the toxoid.

Which two vaccinations should be given to sickle cell patients as prophylaxis?

1. Haemophilus Influenzae vaccine
2. S. pneumoniae vaccine.
Since sickle cell patients are functionally asplenic and prone to infection from encapsulated organisms.

Which vaccinations are important to be given to elderly patients?

Pneumococcal (>65 years old) and influenza virus (>50 years old) vaccines

Clinical Bacteriology

CHAPTER 6

Gram-Positive Cocci

STAPHYLOCOCCUS

Which enzyme's production differentiates *Staphylococcus* from *Streptococcus*?

Catalase

Mnemonic: Cat-in-A-Staff
(*Staphylococcus aureus*)

Which *Staphylococcus* species forms bubbles when mixed with hydrogen peroxide?

Staphylococcus aureus. Catalase degrades peroxide (H_2O_2) into H_2O and O_2 gas causing bubbles to form.

Describe the appearance of *Staphylococcus* under the microscope:

Gram-positive irregular grapelike clusters

Where is *S. aureus* most often found? Why is this medically important?

Nose. Serves as a reservoir for community- or hospital-acquired methicillin-resistant *S. aureus* (MRSA).

What five features differentiate *S. aureus* from other species of *Staphylococcus*?

1. Coagulase positive
2. Mannitol fermentation
3. β-Hemolytic
4. Protein A
5. Exotoxins

What is protein A and where is it found?

Virulence factor in the cell wall of *S. aureus* that binds to the Fc portion of immunoglobulin G (IgG), preventing activation of complement, opsonization, and phagocytosis

What two other important cell wall virulence factors does *S. aureus* possess?

1. Teichoic acid
2. Polysaccharide capsule

What are the three most clinically important exotoxins produced by *S. aureus*?

1. Enterotoxin
2. Toxic shock syndrome toxin (TSST)
3. Exfoliatin (Scalded skin syndrome)

Which toxin is associated with food poisoning causing vomiting and watery, nonbloody diarrhea? How long do symptoms last? Is it preformed?

Enterotoxin. Food poisoning is self-limited, lasting about 2 hours. Preformed toxin, onset within 4 hours of ingestion.

Which foods are associated with S. aureus food poisoning?

Improperly kept eggs, dairy, meat

Which S. aureus toxin(s) act as a superantigen and what do superantigens do?

Enterotoxin and TSST. Activate a subpopulation of T cells with the Vβ-receptor subtype leading to a massive cytokine response

Which cytokines are released by superantigens and what is the clinical result?

Interleukin-1 (IL-1), interleukin-2 (IL-2), tumor necrosis factor (TNF) leading to systemic shock, disseminated intra-vascular coagulation (DIC), and organ failure (heart and kidney)

What is the mechanism of action of exfoliatin?

Cleaves desmoglein in desmosomes causing separation of the epidermis (the cause of staphylococcal scaled skin syndrome)

What are other important S. aureus exotoxins and their mechanisms of action?

   Coagulase

Activates clotting around S. aureus, thereby preventing phagocytosis

   Staphylokinase

Lyses thrombi and prevents body from "walling-off" an infection

   Hyaluronidase

Lyses the connective tissue matrix facilitating spread

   Hemolysin and leukocidin

Lyses red blood cells (RBCs) (therefore β-hemolytic) and white blood cells (WBCs)

   β-Lactamase

Cleaves penicillin family (i.e., β-lactam) drugs

Mnemonic: Toxins make S. aureus a Body **LEECH** (TSST, Staphylokinase, β-lactamase, Leukocidin, Enterotoxin, Exfoliatin, Coagulase, and Hemolysin/Hyaluronidase)

What are some predisposing factors to infections by S. aureus?

Diabetes, intravenous (IV) drug use, foreign bodies (sutures, IV catheters)

Staphylococcus aureus is the most common cause of postsurgical wound infections. What other skin infections are associated with it?

Impetigo/cellulitis, Furuncles/carbuncles (hair follicle), Mastitis (nursing breasts)

Describe the lesion in impetigo. What patient population presents with impetigo?

Bullae that burst and become *honey crusted*. Seen commonly in children

What is used to treat methicillin-sensitive *S. aureus* infections?

β-Lactamase–resistant penicillin (nafcillin, dicloxacillin) or β-lactam/β-lactamase inhibitor combination

How is methicillin-resistant *S. aureus* (MRSA) treated?

Vancomycin for severe infections. Bactrim, clindamycin, doxycycline for milder infections. Linezolid and daptomycin may also be used as alternatives.

What differentiates *Staphylococcus epidermidis* from *Staphylococcus saprophyticus*?

Novobiocin sensitivity. *Staphylococcus saprophyticus* is the only *Staphylococcus* resistant to novobiocin.

Where is *S. epidermidis* normally found?

Skin and mucous membranes

What are the two typical diseases caused by *S. epidermidis*?

1. Prosthetic valve endocarditis
2. IV catheter infection

What allows adherence by *S. epidermidis* to prosthetic material?

Glycocalyx on its capsule

What type of infection is *S. saprophyticus* associated with?

Second most common cause of urinary tract infections (UTIs) in sexually active younger women. Most common is *Escherichia Coli.*

Mnemonic: drinking **Sapporo** and not **resisting** your **novio** leads to **UTIs**

How do you treat *S. saprophyticus* UTIs?

Fluoroquinolones or trimethoprim-sulfamethoxazole (TMP-SMX)

STREPTOCOCCUS

How are *Streptococcus* species classified?

According to Lancefield group (antigen characteristics of the C carbohydrate found on the cell wall) or type of hemolysis

Describe the Lancefield group, type of hemolysis, and key diagnostic features for the following:

Streptococcus pyogenes

Lancefield group A, β-hemolytic, bacitracin sensitive

Streptococcus agalactiae

Lancefield group B, β-hemolytic, bacitracin resistant

Enterococcus faecalis **and** *Enterococcus faecium*

Lancefield group D, α- or β-hemolytic, growth in 6.5% NaCl

Note that enterococci are no longer considered streptococci.

Streptococcus gallolyticus

Lancefield group D, α-hemolytic, no growth in 6.5% NaCl

Streptococcus pneumoniae

No Lancefield group, α-hemolytic, bile soluble, inhibited by optochin

Viridans group streptococci

No Lancefield group, α-hemolytic, not bile soluble, not inhibited by optochin

What virulence factor causes β-hemolysis?

Streptolysin O and S. Streptolysin O is inactivated by oxygen and antistreptolysin O (ASO) antibodies are important in the diagnosis of rheumatic fever. Streptolysin S is oxygen stable and is not immunogenic.

What is M protein?

Antiphagocytic virulence factor *S. pyogenes*. Specific types of M protein are associated with pharyngitis/acute rheumatic fever, cellulitis/acute glomerulonephritis, and necrotizing fasciitis. The body makes antibodies against the M protein.

What toxins are associated with *S. pyogenes*?

Erythrogenic toxin, exotoxins A and B, streptolysin O and S

Which toxins act as superantigens?

Erythrogenic and exotoxin A

Which one is more often associated with streptococcal toxic shock syndrome (TSS)?

Exotoxin A causes more cases of TSS.

Through what three broad pathogenic mechanisms do *Streptococcus pyogenes* cause disease?

1. Pyogenic inflammation (pharyngitis and cellulitis)
2. Toxin-mediated diseases (scarlet fever, toxic shock syndrome)
3. Immunologic diseases/delayed antibody-mediated diseases (rheumatic fever and glomerulonephritis)

How does *S. pyogenes* pharyngitis usually present and why must it be treated with antibiotics?

High fevers, pharyngeal erythema, swollen tonsils with exudates, and tender cervical lymph nodes. It should be treated with penicillin or a cephalosporin because untreated infections may result in rheumatic fever.

Why is it always important to treat *Streptococcus* impetigo? What complication only arises from *Streptococcus* pharyngitis and not *Streptococcus* impetigo?

Glomerulonephritis may develop secondary to untreated *Streptococcus* impetigo. Rheumatic fever only develops after *Streptococcus* pharyngitis infections.

What is necrotizing fasciitis and how is it treated?

Very serious subcutaneous infection that spreads rapidly along fascial plane typically after trauma of the skin. Can be either polymicrobial or monomicrobial (classically *S. pyogenes*). Treat with aggressive surgical debridement (including amputation) and antibiotics active against the likely pathogens. (If group A *Streptococcus*, use penicillin and clindamycin. Clindamycin is added because it helps to inhibit toxin production.)

What is rheumatic fever?

Immunologic disease caused by cross-reactivity of *S. pyogenes* M protein and antigens of joint and heart tissue. Clinically it presents 2–3 weeks following *S. pyogenes* pharyngitis (strep throat) and manifests with fever, migratory arthritis, chorea (rapid purposeless movements), carditis (new-onset murmur), subcutaneous nodules, and erythema marginatum (rash with pale centers and red margins).

Mnemonic: JONES = Joints, O as a heart symbol for pancarditis, Nodules, Erythema marginatum, Sydenham's chorea (rapid jerking movements)

Pathology Correlate: What are the pathognomonic lesions of rheumatic heart disease?

Aschoff bodies, which are foci of fibrinoid necrosis surrounded by lymphocytes and macrophages known as Anitschkow cells.

How is rheumatic fever diagnosed?

Using the modified Jones criteria, which require two major criteria (carditis, migratory polyarthritis, subcutaneous nodules, erythema marginatum, chorea) or one major plus two minor criteria (previous history of acute rheumatic fever, elevated C-reactive protein, ASO titer)

Where is the most frequent damaged site of the heart as a result of recurrent infections with streptococci?

Mitral valve is the most common site followed by the aortic valve. The damaged valve may be apparent after many years as a heart murmur on physical examination. Prolonged penicillin therapy for prophylaxis is required to prevent future infections with *S. pyogenes*. Once heart valves are damaged, patients should be given amoxicillin before any dental or surgical procedure.

What is poststreptococcal acute glomerulonephritis (AGN)?

Immunologic disease caused by deposited antigen-antibody complexes onto the glomerular basement membrane leading to glomerular destruction. Clinically it presents 2–3 weeks after *S. pyogenes* cellulitis or pharyngitis with hypertension, edema, and urine with RBC casts, oliguria, and azotemia.

Describe the immunofluorescence pattern of AGN glomerular basement membranes. What complement factor is decreased in the serum as a result?

Immune complexes form, resulting in granular subepithelial deposits referred to as "humps" or "lumpy bumpy." C3 is decreased.

What is scarlet fever?

Erythrogenic toxin-mediated disease that develops in association with infections of certain strains of *S. pyogenes* and is characterized by a course, erythematous, blanching rash; a strawberry tongue; petechial lesions in skin creases (Pastia sign); and desquamation of the skin. The erythrogenic toxin is acquired by lysogenic conversion.

What diseases are associated with group B streptococci or *S. agalactiae*?

Sepsis and meningitis in neonates and UTIs (some women may have vaginal colonization by *S. agalactiae* and infect the baby during vaginal delivery), soft tissue, and endocarditis infections in adults

What diseases are associated with group D *Enterococcus* (*E. faecalis* and *E. faecium*)?

UTIs, endocarditis, biliary tree infection, and peritonitis

What type of cancer is associated with non-*Enterococcus* group D *Streptococcus* (*S. bovis*)?

Colon cancer

What Streptococci have no Lancefield group and are alpha-hemolytic?

S. pneumoniae and viridans group streptococci

What are the viridans group streptococci and where are they normally found?

Human gastrointestinal tract flora. They are normally found in the nasopharynx and gingival crevices. Usually associated with dental infections (*Streptococcus mutans*), subacute bacterial endocarditis (heart valve destruction), and abscesses (*Streptococcus intermedius* group). Order a CT scan with contrast to detect an abscess in the body if *S. intermedius* is extracted from the blood.

What diseases do *S. pneumonia* cause?

MOPS: Meningitis meningitis (most common cause of bacterial meningitis in adults), otitis media (most common cause in children), pneumonia, sinusitis

How is *S. pneumoniae* described under the microscope?

Gram-positive lancet-shaped diplococci

What are the important virulence factors for *S. pneumoniae*?

Polysaccharide capsule, IgA protease, pneumolysin, and lipotechoic acid

What is the clinical significance of the polysaccharide capsule?

It is antiphagocytic, antibodies to the capsule are protective (*S. pneumoniae* vaccine). Asplenic patients (associated with decreased opsonin antibody production) are more susceptible to severe *S. pneumoniae* infections.

What is the clinical significance of the IgA protease?

IgA protease allows for infection of the respiratory tract, leading to sinusitis and lobar pneumonia (with characteristic "rusty-colored" sputum).

How is *S. pneumoniae* treated?

Although penicillin is the drug of choice, penicillin resistance is increasingly prevalent by virtue of altered penicillin-binding proteins.

Who should receive the *S. pneumonia* vaccine?

Older patients (>65), immunocompromised patients, diabetics, asplenic patients, and chronic obstructive pulmonary disease (COPD) patients

CLINICAL VIGNETTES

A previously healthy young woman was admitted to the intensive care unit (ICU) with high fever, hypotension, nausea, vomiting, disseminated sunburn-like rash, generalized muscle ache, and imminent cardiac and renal failure. Her last menstrual period was about 5 days ago. What is the most likely diagnosis?

Toxic shock syndrome, most likely secondary to *S. aureus* from tampon use

A preschooler presents with a superficial skin infection characterized by erythema with pustules and a honey-colored crust. There are areas of superficial bullae, and some have ruptured leaving raw exudative areas. What is the diagnosis and what are the causative organisms?

Impetigo. *Staphylococcus aureus* more commonly than group A *Streptococcus*

A 3-month-old male infant presents with extensive bullae and areas of denuded skin, with the epidermis easily dislodging under pressure. His mother had a recent bacterial infection. What is the diagnosis and causative organism?

Scalded skin syndrome caused by staphylococcal exotoxin

A child presents with a rash that is diffusely erythematous, with superimposed fine red papules, and is most pronounced in the groin and axilla. His face is notably flushed and he has *strawberry tongue* (enlarged red papillae coating the tongue). Prior to the rash, he had a sore throat. What is your presumed diagnosis?

Scarlet fever caused by erythrogenic toxin of *S. pyogenes*

A boy presents with sore throat, arthralgias, headache, and fever. On examination, his tonsils are enlarged, erythematous, and covered with white exudates. He also has tender cervical lymphadenopathy. You diagnose the patient with pharyngitis and swab his throat to look for organism on culture. What are two feared complications from this infection?

Group A streptococci (*S. pyogenes*)
1. Poststreptococcal glomerulonephritis
2. Rheumatic fever

A 55-year-old woman develops Janeway lesions, Osler nodes, splinter hemorrhages, and Roth spots about 1 month after a tooth extraction. She has a history of rheumatic heart disease. What is the most common causative microbe?

This patient has infective endocarditis. Viridans group *Streptococcus* is the most common cause of subacute infective endocarditis, while *S. aureus* is the most common cause of acute infective endocarditis.

CHAPTER 7

Gram-Positive Rods

Do all *Bacillus* bacteria form spores?	Yes
What other gram-positive rods form endospores?	*Clostridium* species also form spores.
Which gram-positive rods don't form spores?	*Corynebacterium* and *Listeria*

BACILLUS ANTHRACIS

Name three pathologic manifestations of *Bacillus anthracis* and their routes of transmission:	1. Cutaneous anthrax by contact with animal products contaminated with spores 2. Pulmonary anthrax (or woolsorter's disease) by direct inhalation of spores 3. Gastrointestinal anthrax by indigestion of contaminated meat **Mnemonic: P**athogenic **S**pores Germinate (**P**ulmonary, **S**kin [cutaneous], gastrointestinal [**GI**])
Name the three virulence factors of *B. anthracis* and describe their mechanism of action:	1. Capsule is antiphagocytic. 2. Edema factor exotoxin is acalmodulin-dependent adenylate cyclase that increases cyclic adenosine monophosphate (cAMP) causing severe edema. 3. Lethal factor exotoxin is a protease, causing cells to increase tumor necrosis factor (TNF) production leading to cell death.
What is the importance of the protective antigen?	Virulence factors must be paired with the protective antigen to express toxicity.

What are the clinical symptoms of cutaneous anthrax? What is the overall mortality rate?

Painless papules that evolve into vesicles and then necrotic black eschar over the course of several days, then spreading to lymph nodes and blood, resulting in sepsis if untreated. Mortality rate of 20%.

What are the clinical symptoms of pulmonary anthrax? What is the overall mortality rate?

First stage (first 2–3 days) consists of influenza-like symptoms such as dry cough, fever, and aches. Then sudden progression to second stage, which is characterized by difficulty breathing, substernal pressure due to bloody pleural effusion, and sepsis. Chest x-ray shows widening of the mediastinum. Mortality rate near 100% if untreated.

What are the clinical symptoms of gastrointestinal anthrax? What is the overall mortality rate?

Bloody vomiting, bloody diarrhea, abdominal pain, fever. Mortality rate of 25%–60%

How is anthrax usually treated?

Penicillin, tetracyclines, and fluoroquinolones

BACILLUS CEREUS

Name the most common clinical association with *Bacillus cereus*:

Food poisoning from reheated rice

Name the two toxins made by *B. cereus*.

1. Heat-labile toxin
2. Heat-stable toxin

Name the gram-negative rod that produces a toxin similar to the heat-labile toxin of *B. cereus*. What are their mechanisms of action?

Vibrio cholerae cholera toxin. Both toxins trigger adenosine diphosphate (ADP)-ribosylation of G protein, stimulating adenylate cyclase and increasing cAMP. (ADP-ribosylation is a common mechanism used by various bacterial toxins.) Increased cAMP triggers massive efflux of water and ions from infected enterocytes resulting in profuse watery diarrhea.

What are the clinical symptoms caused by the heat-labile and heat-stable toxins?

Rapid onset (<5 hours) of vomiting and nausea following ingestion of food is classic for heat-stable toxin. Onset of voluminous, watery, nonbloody diarrhea, nausea, vomiting, and abdominal pain after an incubation period up to 16 hours is characteristic of heat-labile toxin.

How is *B. cereus* treated?

The food poisoning is self-limited, so it is treated with supportive care to prevent dehydration.

CLOSTRIDIUM BOTULINUM

Do *Clostridium* species require oxygen?

No, they are all obligate anaerobes.

What diseases does *C. botulinum* cause?

Clostridium botulinum causes foodborne botulism (ingestion of preformed toxin), infant botulism (ingestion of spores that germinate in gut-producing toxins), and wound botulism (injection of spores that germinate in tissue-producing toxins).

What is the mechanism of botulinum toxin in causing botulism?

The toxin blocks the release of acetylcholine (Ach), resulting in flaccid paralysis.

What usually causes infant botulism? What are its associated symptoms?

Results from infant ingestion of contaminated honey leading to lethargy, and decreased muscle tone, *floppy baby syndrome*; most common type of botulism in the United States

What are the symptoms of classic botulism?

Cranial paralysis, including diplopia, ptosis, dysphagia, symmetric, **descending motor paralysis**, and death due to respiratory failure

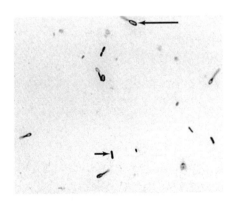

Figure 7.1 Terminal spores on Clostridium demonstrated on Gram stain. (*With permission from Brooks GF, Carroll KC, Butel JS, & Morse SA. Jawetz, Melnick & Adelberg's Medical Microbiology. 24th ed. New York, NY: McGraw-Hill; 2007.*)

How is botulism treated?

Classic botulism can be treated with respiratory care and antitoxin; as for infant botulism, infants typically recover spontaneously with supportive care.

CLOSTRIDIUM DIFFICILE

Name the most common disease associated with *Clostridium difficile*:

Pseudomembranous colitis

What commonly causes pseudomembranous colitis?

Usage of broad-spectrum antibiotic treatment (e.g., clindamycin or ampicillin) results in suppression of normal GI flora and proliferation of *C. difficile*. *Clostridium difficile* is usually acquired from the hospital environment.

Name the two exotoxins produced by *C. difficile*:

1. Cytotoxin (toxin B)
2. Enterotoxin (toxin A)

Which one of the two exotoxins produced by *C. difficile* is most responsible for pseudomembranous colitis?

Cytotoxin (toxin B) kills enterocytes causing pseudomembrane formation.

How is pseudomembranous colitis treated?

Discontinue offending drug and start oral vancomycin. Metronidazole is classically given but no longer considered first-line therapy. Both suppress *C. difficile* and allow normal flora to return. Fidaxomicin, fecal microbiota transplants, and bowel transplants are reserved as secondary treatment.

CLOSTRIDIUM PERFRINGENS

Name the conditions most often associated with *Clostridium perfringens*:

Myonecrosis (gas gangrene), cellulitis, food poisoning, necrotizing enteritis

Name two major toxins by *C. perfringens*:

1. α-Toxin (lecithinase)
2. Enterotoxin (heat-labile toxin)

What is the role of α toxin in myonecrosis?

α-Toxin lyses red blood cells, endothelial cells, leukocytes, and platelets. This facilitates invasion of muscles near the infected wounds, leading to the production of subcutaneous gas (hence the name gas gangrene).

How is gas gangrene treated?	Surgical debridement of necrotic tissue, antibiotics (penicillin plus clindamycin), and hyperbaric oxygen chamber may disrupt anaerobic progression of myonecrosis.
How does *C. perfringens* food poisoning usually present?	Abdominal cramps, diarrhea, and fever that presents 8 to 18 hours after ingestion of contaminated beef, poultry, pork, and fish. It takes more time than *Staphylococcus aureus* to develop symptoms because *C. perfringens* has to grow and produce enterotoxin in vivo.
How is *C. perfringens* food poisoning treated?	Supportive care treatment because it is a self-limiting disease

CLOSTRIDIUM TETANI

How does *Clostridium tetani* cause tetanus?	*Clostridium tetani* acquired from traumatic wound releases tetanus toxin (exotoxin), which blocks the release of inhibitory neurotransmitter glycine and γ-aminobutyric acid (GABA) from Renshaw cells in spinal cord.
What are the symptoms of tetanus? Why?	Spastic paralysis due to prolonged muscle contracture results from lack of inhibition (i.e., loss of glycine), resulting in dysphagia (early), trismus (lockjaw), risus sardonicus (grimace), and respiratory failure.
How is tetanus treated?	Antitoxin, antibiotics, sedatives, and muscle relaxants to prevent spasms, and debridement of wound
What is the tetanus vaccine made of?	Formalin-inactivated tetanus toxoid
What is in a diphtheria, tetanus, and pertussis (DTaP) childhood vaccine?	Diphtheria toxin, tetanus toxoid, and acellular pertussis antigen

CORYNEBACTERIUM DIPHTHERIAE

Does *Corynebacterium diphtheria* **form spores or have a capsule?**

No, it is nonspore forming and nonencapsulated.

What disease is caused by *C. diphtheriae?* **Name its typical symptoms:**

Diphtheria. Lymphadenopathy (bull neck) and pseudomembrane pharyngitis (i.e., thick, gray exudative pseudomembrane in the throat and nasopharynx)

How is *C. diphtheriae* **transmitted?**

Via airborne droplets

How is *C. diphtheriae's* **exotoxin encoded?**

β-Prophage DNA

What is exotoxin's mechanism of action?

ADP ribosylation of elongation factor-2 (EF-2) blocks tRNA translocation causing inhibition of host protein synthesis.

What are the major complications of diphtheria?

Physical airway obstruction, myocarditis, demyelination/paralysis of peripheral nerves

Mnemonic: Diphtheria affects **MAN** (**M**yocarditis, **A**irway, **N**erves).

What type of agar is used for culturing *C. diphtheriae?*

Tinsdale potassium tellurite agar

How is *C. diphtheriae* **diagnosed?**

Laboratory diagnosis is based on grampositive rods with metachromatic (blue and red) granules.

How is diphtheria treated? Prevented?

Immediate administration of horse serum antitoxin, then antibiotics (penicillin G and erythromycin), and then vaccine in that order. Prevented with **diphtheria, tetanus, and acellular pertussis** (DTaP) vaccine

LISTERIA MONOCYTOGENES

Describe the morphology and special characteristics of *Listeria*:	Small gram-positive bacillus, facultative intracellular, β-hemolysis, catalase positive, tumbling motility at room temperature
What is unique about the growth characteristic of *Listeria*?	It grows well in cold temperature (4°C–10°C).
What is the most prominent virulence factor in *Listeria*? How does it work?	Listeriolysin O toxin penetrates host cell's phagocytic vacuole to facilitate bacterial entry into the cytoplasm.
What is unique about the mechanism in which *Listeria* infects cells?	*Listeria* has the ability to spread from cell to cell without entering the extracellular environment by using an actin polymerization propulsion system called "actin rockets."
What type of motility does *Listeria* display?	Tumbling motility
What diseases are caused by *Listeria*?	Meningoencephalitis, sepsis, infections in pregnancy (leading to premature birth or fetal death), and gastroenteritis are the most common manifestations of *Listeria*.
What patient populations are typically affected by *Listeria monocytogenes*? Why?	Pregnant women, newborns of infected mothers, elderly, and immunosuppressed patients. *Listeria* is a facultative intracellular organism and requires an intact cell-mediated immunity to clear.
How is *Listeria* transmitted?	Most commonly via unpasteurized dairy, meats, and vegetables. Also, transplacental spread during delivery
How is *Listeria* treated?	Ampicillin (with gentamicin for serious cases or trimethoprim-sulfamethoxazole for penicillin-allergic patients). *Listeria* is always resistant to cephalosporins.

CLINICAL VIGNETTES

A 43-year-old man who has been taking amoxicillin for 3 weeks to treat an upper respiratory tract infection suddenly develops low-grade fever and diarrhea. What has he most likely developed, which pathogen is causing his new symptoms, and what is the treatment of choice?

He has developed pseudomembranous colitis from overgrowth of C. *difficile* due to broad-spectrum antibiotic therapy. Treat with metronidazole and stop the amoxicillin.

Spores of this bacterium enter the body through a traumatic wound, causing pain, edema, and cellulitis. Degenerative enzymes produce gas in tissues, evident by crepitation. Hemolysis, jaundice, and bloody exudates are common. Mortality rates are high. What is the causative organism and disease?

Clostridium perfringens causing gas gangrene (myonecrosis), early surgical debridement, antibiotics (penicillin, clindamycin), and hyperbaric oxygen

A young girl presents with fever, sore throat, and regurgitating fluids through her nose. Physical examination reveals cervical lymphadenopathy and a thick, gray, adherent pseudomembrane over the tonsils and throat, and paralysis of the soft palate. What is the likely diagnosis and causative organism?

Diphtheria caused by C. *diphtheriae*

A 55-year-old drum-maker presents with nonspecific respiratory symptoms, low-grade fever, and substernal discomfort. Chest x-ray reviews a widening mediastinum. What is the likely diagnosis?

"Woolsorter's disease" or inhalational anthrax caused by B. *anthracis*, a life-threatening pneumonia, which can progress from nonspecific respiratory symptoms to hemorrhagic mediastinitis, bloody pleural effusions, septic shock, and death

CHAPTER 8

Gram-Negative Cocci (Neisseria)

What is the characteristic appearance of both *Neisseria gonorrhoeae* and *Neisseria meningitidis* under the microscope?

Gram-negative kidney-shaped diplococci

Describe the sugar fermentation patterns of *N. gonorrhoeae* and *N. meningitidis*:

N. gonorrhoeae ferments only glucose whereas *N. meningitidis* ferments both glucose and maltose.

What enzyme common to both *N. gonorrhoeae* and *N. meningitides* allows them to colonize mucosal surfaces? Which gram-positive organism also shares this enzyme.

IgA protease. *S. pneumoniae*

NEISSERIA GONORRHOEAE

Name the most common pathologic manifestations of infection by *N. gonorrhoeae*:

Purulent urethritis, cervicitis, epididymitis, pelvic inflammatory disease, neonatal conjunctivitis, disseminated gonococcal infection (two forms: tenosynovitis and skin lesions or septic arthritis most commonly involving the knee)

Which growth media is used for the isolation and identification of *N. gonorrhoeae*?

Thayer-Martin vancomycin, colistin, and nystatin (VCN) media

Name a mechanism by which *N. gonorrhoeae* evades host defenses:

Antigenic and phase variation of its surface proteins (pili)

Is vaginal and penile discharge caused by *N. gonorrhoeae* usually purulent or clear and why?

Purulent due to a neutrophilic exudate

Identification of gram-negative diplococci in urethral discharge within which cell type is sufficient for the diagnosis of gonorrhea in men?	Neutrophils
What are the most common complications in men of gonococcal urethritis?	Epididymitis, prostatitis, urethral strictures
What are the major long-term complications of *N. gonorrhoeae* induced pelvic inflammatory disease?	Sterility, ectopic pregnancy, abscess, peritonitis, perihepatitis (liver capsule)
What complication of pelvic inflammatory disease often caused by *N. gonorrhoeae* involves perihepatitis?	Fitz-Hugh and Curtis syndrome. Patients complain of right upper quadrant pain and tenderness. "Violin strings" adherent to the liver capsule
Describe the key symptoms of both forms of disseminated gonococcal infection.	1. Tenosynovitis, dermatitis, and migratory polyarthralgia. 2. Purulent arthritis with sudden onset mono- or oligoarthritis usually involves distal joints (knee, wrists, and ankles)
How is *N. gonorrhoeae* treated?	Ceftriaxone plus azithromycin. Prophylaxis for neonatal conjunctivitis with silver nitrate (Not commonly used anymore due to chemical conjunctivitis) or erythromycin into both eyes immediately after birth
What other bacterial coinfection must be considered in treating *N. gonorrhoeae* infections?	Chlamydial infection is a common coinfection with gonorrhea, so antibiotic treatment should cover both organisms (add azithromycin or doxycycline). Sexual partners also need to be evaluated for treatment.

NEISSERIA MENINGITIDIS

Name the most important clinical diseases caused by *N. meningitidis*:	Meningitis, meningococcemia (fulminant form: Waterhouse-Friderichsen syndrome)
How does *N. meningitidis* spread? Name one mechanism that allows *N. meningitidis* to escape host defenses:	Spread via respiratory secretions Antiphagocytic polysaccharide capsule
What are the two highest risk groups for *N. meningitidis* infection?	1. Infants 6 months to 2 years (<6 months protected by maternal antibodies) 2. Young adults brought into crowded conditions such as military recruits and college students in dorms or during the Hajj. Frequent epidemics in sub-Saharan Africa
What type of immunodeficiency has the greatest risk of *N. meningitides* bacteremia?	Persons deficient in terminal complement components C6 to C9
What are the key clinical aspects of a patient who leads to a diagnosis of meningococcemia?	Prodrome of fever, headache, nausea followed by vomiting, hypotension, myalgias, discrete pink macules, papules, petechiae distributed over the trunk, extremities, and palate
What virulence factor causes the petechiae seen in meningococcal infections?	Endotoxin-mediated blood vessel destruction leading to blood vessel hemorrhage
What are the key signs of meningitis associated with *N. meningitides* infection?	Fever, nuchal rigidity, vomiting, lethargy, altered mental status. In young children, irritability, seizures, and they may not have nuchal rigidity
What are typical lumbar puncture findings in bacterial meningitis?	Increased intracranial pressure, turbid cerebrospinal fluid (CSF) with greater than 1000 WBC/μL (predominantly polymorphonuclear [PMN]), increased total protein, decreased glucose, and characteristic bacteria on Gram stain

What is Waterhouse-Friderichsen syndrome and what are its most common manifestations?

Fulminant meningococcemia leading to septic shock and bilateral adrenal hemorrhage causing a catastrophic adrenal insufficiency and death in hours

How is *N. meningitidis* spread to close contacts? How can *N. meningitides* infection be prevented in close contacts?

Spread via asymptomatic nasopharyngeal carriers. Contact prophylaxis with rifampin or ciprofloxacin

How are *N. meningitidis* infections prevented?

Purified polysaccharide vaccine for groups A, C, Y, and W135. A conjugate vaccine for those four capsular polysaccharides is also available. Serogroup B vaccine is also available and recommended for high-risk individuals 10 years or older.

What is the treatment of *N. meningitidis* infection?

Penicillin G (it does not eradicate *N. meningitidis* from the nasopharynx) or a cephalosporin with good CNS penetration (e.g., ceftriaxone)

Which part of *N. gonorrhoeae* undergoes antigenic variation making it difficult to completely eradicate or develop a vaccine?

Pili, outer membrane proteins (Opa), lipooligosaccharide (LOS)

CLINICAL VIGNETTES

A 23-year-old college student presents to his school's student health office complaining of painful urination and purulent urethral discharge for the last 3 days. Analysis of the discharge reveals gram-negative diplococci. What is the offending pathogen and what is the treatment of choice?

Neisseria gonorrhoeae, IM ceftriaxone, and azithromycin (Due to presumed coinfection with chlamydia)

A 19-year-old college student presents to the ER with headache, malaise, and fever (102°F). On examination, there is nuchal rigidity and on the lower extremities there are petechiae and purpura. What is the most likely diagnosis?

Meningitis with petechiae is most often associated with meningococcal meningitis.

An 18-year-old woman presents with a sore throat. She is sexually active with a new boyfriend who was recently treated for an unknown sexually transmitted disease (STD). What is the most likely diagnosis? How do you diagnose this?

Gonococcal pharyngitis. Diagnose by pharyngeal culture.

CHAPTER 9

Gram-Negative Rods (Enterics)

ESCHERICHIA COLI

Name the common diseases caused by *Escherichia coli*:

Escherichia coli can cause diarrhea (bloody and nonbloody), urinary tract infections (UTIs) (most common cause), neonatal meningitis (second most common after group B *streptococci*), gram-negative sepsis (most common cause), and nosocomial pneumonia.

Where does *E. coli* normally colonize and how is it transmitted?

Escherichia coli is considered normal flora of the colon that is transmitted via fecal-oral route.

How is an *E. coli* infection diagnosed?

Laboratory culture. *Escherichia coli* is gram negative, oxidase negative, lactose fermenting, and β-hemolytic (although not all strains are lactose fermenting or β-hemolytic).

What three antigens are classically associated with *Escherichia coli*? Which two are commonly used for serology?

1. O antigen (somatic antigen)
2. K antigen (capsular antigen)
3. H antigen (flagellar antigen)
O and H are used for serology.

What larger structure is the O antigen a part of?

O antigen is part of lipopolysaccharide (LPS) (endotoxin).

What does the lack of H antigen signify?

H antigen is part of the flagellae. Strains without it lack flagellae and are nonmotile.

Why would *E. coli* with the K1 antigen be troubling to physicians?	K1 strains cause neonatal meningitis, bacteremia, and urinary tract infection.
What are five strains of virulent enteric *E. coli*?	1. Enterotoxigenic *E. coli* (ETEC) 2. Enterohemorrhagic *E. coli* (EHEC) 3. Enteroinvasive *E. coli* (EIEC) 4. Enteropathogenic *E. coli* (EPEC) 5. Enteroaggregative *E. coli* (EAEC)
What two toxins does ETEC *traveler's diarrhea* produce?	1. Heat-labile toxin (LT) 2. Heat-stable toxin (ST)
What is the mechanism of heat LT?	Constitutively activates Gs via adenosine diphosphate (ADP) ribosylation leading to constant activation of adenylate cyclase and high levels of cyclic adenosine monophosphate (cAMP). This causes increased secretion of Cl– ions from intestinal cells into the gastrointestinal (GI) lumen. Negative Cl– ions cause positively charged Na+ ions to follow. Water follows Na+ into the lumen leading to diarrhea.
What is the mechanism of action for ST?	Constitutively activates guanylate cyclase leading to increased cyclic guanosine monophosphate (cGMP) and ultimately decreased water absorption from the GI lumen
Which other bacterial toxin is similar to LT toxin?	Cholera toxin
What toxin mediates EHEC diarrhea? What is the mechanism of action?	Shiga-like toxin (verocytotoxin) inhibits 28S component of the 60S ribosome subunit, inhibiting protein synthesis leading to cell necrosis of the intestinal epithelium and hemorrhagic colitis. **Mnemonic: Shiga**-like it's the 19**60s**
How do patients with EHEC present?	Afebrile and bloody diarrhea without inflammatory white blood cells. EHEC strain O157:H7 is associated with hemolytic uremic syndrome (HUS)
What is the mechanism that causes hemolytic uremic syndrome (HUS)? What are the features of HUS?	HUS occurs when Shiga-like toxin (verocytotoxin) enters the blood stream and damages the vascular endothelium. Cardinal features include thrombocytopenia, anemia, and acute renal failure. **Mnemonic:** You can get HUS from a **RAT** (**R**enal failure, **A**nemia, **T**hrombocytopenia)

How are patients typically exposed to EHEC O157:H7?	Undercooked hamburger meat and direct contact with animals (child presents following a petting zoo visit)
How is EHEC treated?	Fluids and supportive therapy. Antibiotics are not useful and may predispose to HUS.
What other diarrhea causing bacteria are encoded by a plasmid shared in the main virulence factors of EIEC?	*Shigella*
How do these plasmid-encoded proteins act?	These plasmid-encoded proteins allow for adherence and direct invasion of epithelial cells in the gut. Note that this is not toxin-mediated like ETEC and EHEC.
How do patients with EIEC present?	Fever and bloody diarrhea with inflammatory white blood cells (compare to EHEC)
EPEC adheres to but does not invade intestinal cells and results in flattening of the intestinal villi. What is the consequence of this and how does it present?	Flattening of the villi leads to malabsorption. Patients present with fever and bloody diarrhea.
Who does EPEC commonly affect?	Children, associated with nursery breakouts
***Escherichia coli* is the most common cause of UTIs, what is the key virulence factor?**	P-pili that mediate adhesion to urinary epithelium
What finding on urinalysis suggests *E. Coli* infection?	Positive nitrites

SALMONELLA AND *SHIGELLA*

***Salmonella* and *Shigella* are the two important gram-negative bacteria that do not ferment lactose and cause enterocolitis. How are they differentiated?**	*Salmonella* produces gas from glucose fermentation, produces H2S, and is motile (can disseminate hematogenously) **Mnemonic: Salmon** require energy (**glucose**) to swim (**motile**) and smell bad (**H2S**)

Which is more virulent, *Salmonella* or *Shigella*?

Shigella. Less than ten organisms are required for *Shigella* to cause infection because it is very resistant to stomach acid. *Salmonella* is not as resistant and requires 10^6 to 10^9 organisms to cause disease.

What other bacteria besides *Shigella* contain the Shiga toxin?

The hemorrhagic and invasive strains of *E. coli*

What are the mechanisms of the two subunits of Shiga toxin?

Subunit A: Inhibits 60S ribosome, stopping protein synthesis, killing the intestinal cell
Subunit B: Helps subunit A enter cells by binding to the microvillus membrane in the large intestine

What are the reservoirs for *Shigella*?

Only humans, there are no animal carriers

Why does *Shigella* only cause superficial ulcers and not invade blood vessels?

Once *Shigella* enters M cells in the intestine, it uses actin tails to travel among cells without entering the extracellular matrix and remains contained only within the epithelial intestinal cells.

Why is *Shigella* nonmotile?

It lacks the H antigen that codes for motility.

What symptoms are often seen with shigellosis?

Dysentery, bloody diarrhea, fever, and lower abdominal cramps

How is *Shigella* transmitted?

Four Fs: fingers, food, flies, feces

What populations are most often affected by *Shigella*?

Nursing home residents and very young children (ages 2–4 years), especially those in developing countries

What is the treatment of *Shigella* and what medications should be avoided?

Treatment includes fluid/electrolyte replacement and antibiotics such as trimethoprim-sulfamethoxazole (TMP-SMX) and ciprofloxacin. Antidiarrhea medications such as loperamide can prolong illness or worsen the severity and should be avoided.

Are *Salmonella* species divided into typhoidal or nontyphoidal types?

Typhoidal: *Salmonella typhi* and *Salmonella paratyphi* cause typhoid fever.

Describe the diseases caused by each and the species included in each:

Nontyphoidal: *Salmonella enteritidis* and *Salmonella choleraesuis* cause enterocolitis, osteomyelitis, and septicemia.

How do typhoidal strains differ from nontyphoidal strains of *Salmonella* in terms of reservoirs?

Salmonella typhi and *S. paratyphi* have only human reservoirs, while nonty-phoidal strains have both human and animal reservoirs (chickens and turtles).

What makes *S. typhi* resistant to macrophage killing?

Inhibits phagolysosome fusion and defensins resist O_2-dependent and inde-pendent killing.

Where does infection with *S. typhi* begin and where does it spread to?

Salmonella typhi begins in the ileocecal intestine and spreads hematogenously and through the lymphatic system to the liver, bone marrow, gallbladder, and spleen.

What organ harbors *S. typhi* in a chronic carrier state?

Gallbladder (remember Typhoid Mary)

What cells in particular harbor *S. typhi* and facilitate its dissemination?

Monocytes, those in Peyer patches in the ileocecal intestines are the initial target

Typhoid fever is a protracted disease of about 3 weeks. Describe the pathogen-esis and symptoms seen in each week:

Week 1

Bacteremia with fever/chills

Week 2

Monocyte involvement with organ inflammation, abdominal pain, and rash

Week 3

Ulceration of Peyer patches, intestinal bleeding, and shock

Describe the location and appearance of the rash seen in week 2:

Rose spots, small, transient, pink rash located on the abdomen (seen in 30% of patients)

What is the appropriate therapy for *S. typhi* infection?

Ciprofloxacin, ceftriaxone, or azithromycin

What disease is typhoid fever often mistaken for? Why?

Appendicitis, patients present with right lower quadrant abdominal pain without rash.

What are some sources of *Salmonella*?

Undercooked poultry, meat, eggs, greens

How does nontyphoidal *Salmonella* cause enterocolitis and describe the type of diarrhea?

Salmonella directly invades epithelial cells of the small and large intestines. Presents with fever and bloody diarrhea with inflammatory white blood cells (similar to EIEC).

How do you treat *Salmonella* enterocolitis?

Fluid/electrolyte replacement as the disease resolves within a week.

Do you treat *Salmonella* enterocolitis with antibiotics?

No. Antibiotics only prolong disease course.

What patients are at increased risk for *Salmonella* osteomyelitis and sepsis?

Sickle cell disease patients due to functional asplenia

VIBRIO

Describe the characteristic appearance of *Vibrio cholerae*:

Gram-negative rod with a single polar flagellum, giving it a *comma shape*

What does *V. cholerae* require in order to cause the clinical disease cholera?

Infection of *V. cholerae* with the CTX phage that encodes the cholera toxin

How is *V. cholerae* classified?

Classified serologically by the O antigen of its lipopolysaccharide. There are over 200 serogroups but only serogroups O1 and O139 have been associated with large scale epidemics

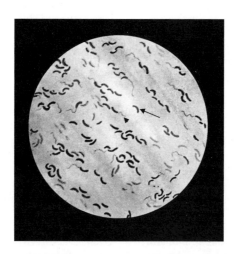

Figure 9.1   Gram stain of *Vibrio cholerae* (long arrow: comma shape; arrow head: flagellum). (*With permission from Levinson WE.* Review of Medical Microbiology and Immunology. *10th ed. New York, NY: McGraw-Hill; 2008.*)

What is the mechanism of action of cholera toxin?

Constitutively activates Gs via ADP ribosylation leading to constant activation of adenylate cyclase and high levels of cAMP. This causes increased secretion of Cl^- ions from intestinal cells into the GI lumen followed by positively charged Na^+ ions. Water follows Na^+ into the lumen leading to watery diarrhea (recall ETEC LT).

What are the physical findings in an individual infected with *V. cholerae*?

Severe dehydration from continuous watery diarrhea with a *rice water* appearance. Look for sunken eyes, poor skin turgor (*skin tenting*), and diminished pulses.

What is the relationship between cholera and stomach acid?

Vibrio cholerae is acid-sensitive; therefore, individuals taking medications to reduce stomach acid (e.g., proton pump inhibitors) may be at increased risk for cholera.

How are *V. cholerae* infections treated?

Rehydration with intravenous (IV) fluid and electrolytes. In milder cases, treat with oral rehydration with electrolyte and glucose solution (e.g., WHO oral rehydration solution). Antibiotics such as doxycycline, tetracycline, and ciprofloxacin may shorten the duration of the illness.

How is *Vibrio parahaemolyticus* transmitted and what are its symptoms?

Vibrio parahaemolyticus is transmitted by ingestion of undercooked seafood (shrimp, sushi, and the like) and is a frequent cause of seafood-associated diarrhea.

How is *Vibrio vulnificus* transmitted and what are its symptoms?

Direct inoculation of contaminated brackish water causes necrotizing wound infections (hand injuries related to opening oysters). Ingestion of raw shellfish causes gastroenteritis and sepsis with necrotizing skin lesions.

Which groups of patients are especially sensitive to *V. vulnificus* septicemia?

Cirrhotic and immunocompromised patients are very susceptible (>40% mortality rate).

CAMPYLOBACTER

Describe the morphology of *Campylobacter*?	*Corkscrew* shaped with long bipolar flagellae. Similar to *Helicobacter pylori*, its specialized shape helps drill through mucous membranes.
What is the clinical progression of disease in an individual infected with *Campylobacter jejuni*?	After incubation of approximately 3 days, patients usually present with abdominal pain and diarrhea. However, approximately one-third of patients present with an influenza-like prodrome (i.e., fever, malaise), followed a day later by severe loose, watery, or bloody stools.
What are the common sources of *C. jejuni* and how is it transmitted?	Poultry (infrequently red meats) and in many domestic animals. Commonly transmitted via cross-contamination (e.g., unwashed cutting board)
What is the most common cause of bloody diarrhea in the United States?	*Campylobacter*
What neurological disorder is associated with *C. jejuni* infection? What is the most concerning aspect of this disorder?	Guillain-Barré syndrome, an autoimmune, demyelinating **ascending** motor paralysis. Most concerning for respiratory failure.
How do you treat *C. jejuni* infection?	Azithromycin. Fluoroquinolone may be suitable alternative if susceptible.

HELICOBACTER PYLORI

What disorder does *H. pylori* most commonly cause?	Duodenal ulcers. Ninety percent of duodenal ulcers are associated with *H. pylori*. (Chronic nonsteroidal anti-inflammatory drug [NSAID] use accounts for the other 10%.)
How can *H. pylori* be biochemically characterized?	Catalase positive, oxidase positive, and urease positive. Urease, an important pathogenic factor, produces ammonia and bicarbonate that neutralizes gastric acids.

How is *H. pylori* diagnosed?

Invasive (endoscopy with biopsy) or noninvasive (serology or urease breath test in which patients drink C14-labeled urea which is then hydrolyzed to ammonia and labeled CO2 that is detected in their breath)

What are the long-term consequences of *H. pylori* infection?

Chronic gastritis, gastric adenocarcinoma, and mucosa-associated lymphoid tumor (MALT) type B-cell lymphoma

What is the combination of medications used to treat *H. pylori* infection?

Triple therapy originally included bismuth salts, metronidazole, and either ampicillin or tetracycline. The current regimen of choice is a proton pump inhibitor, amoxicillin, and clarithromycin.

BACTEROIDES

Bacteroides fragilis is normal colonic flora, but under what conditions does it cause disease?

Bacteroides fragilis has very low virulence; however, intestinal perforation may lead to secondary peritonitis and abscess formation. *Bacteroides fragilis* may also be pathogenic in situations of gyn pathology (pelvic inflammatory disease [PID], septic abortion). Note that 1° peritonitis = spontaneous bacterial peritonitis, 2° = peritonitis due to perforation/necrosis

What is given as antimicrobial prophylaxis prior to abdominal surgery to prevent pathologic infection with *B. fragilis* among other GI pathogens?

Used to be anti-anaerobic cephalosporins or oral metronidazole, but these have largely been replaced by ertapenem

CLINICAL VIGNETTES

A 10-year-old girl with sickle cell disease presents with left knee pain, leukocytosis, and an increased erythrocyte sedimentation rate (ESR). What is the most likely diagnosis and what pathogen is most likely responsible?

Osteomyelitis caused by *Salmonella*

A 30-year-old man presents with fever, abdominal cramps, and watery diarrhea after consuming raw oysters on the prior day. On stool examination, there are RBCs and WBCs. What is the most likely diagnosis?

Vibrio parahaemolyticus

A 15-year-old girl presents with abdominal pain and diarrhea after eating a hamburger at a barbeque the day before. She is afebrile but on rectal examination there is gross blood. Stool analysis is positive for RBCs and negative for fecal leukocytes. What is the most likely diagnosis? How do you confirm the diagnosis? What is a possible sequela of this infection?

Enterohemorrhagic *E. coli* O157:H7. Confirm with stool culture. May lead to hemolytic uremic syndrome (HUS)

CHAPTER 10

Gram-Negative Rods (Respiratory)

Name the five medically important respiratory gram-negative rods:	1. *Klebsiella* 2. *Bordetella* 3. *Legionella* 4. *Haemophilus* 5. *Pseudomonas* **Mnemonic: K**eep **B**reathing a **L**ittle **H**arder **P**lease (*Klebsiella*, *Bordetella*, *Legionella*, *Haemophilus*, *Pseudomonas*)

HAEMOPHILUS INFLUENZAE

Name the diseases caused by *Haemophilus influenzae*:	Bronchitis, sinusitis, pneumonia, otitis media, conjunctivitis, epiglottitis, bacterial meningitis
What other organisms should be in the differential when considering *H. influenzae* infection of the head and neck?	*Moraxella catarrhalis* and *Streptococcus pneumoniae*
Describe the morphology of *H. influenzae*:	Encapsulated gram-negative pleomorphic coccobacillus
What special culture requirements does *H. influenzae* have?	Chocolate agar with factors V (nicotinamide adenine dinucleotide [NAD]) and X (hematin) Coculture *H. influenzae* with *Staphylococcus aureus* on blood agar because *S. aureus* hemolyzes red blood cells (RBCs) releasing factors V and X.
What does *Haemophilus* mean? (It is a clue to its culture requirements.)	Blood loving

**What are the virulence factors of
H. influenzae?**

Capsule (six serotypes), lipopolysaccharide (LPS), attachment factors (pili,
fibrils, protein *H. influenzae* adhesin
[Hia]), immunoglobulin A (IgA)
protease

**What is unique about capsule serotype
B of *H. influenzae*?**

Associated with invasive infections
in children. B capsule is composed of
repeating polyribosylribitol phosphate
(PRP, pentose sugars); other serotypes
have hexose sugars.

How is *H. influenzae* diagnosed?

Culture in chocolate agar enriched with
NAD (factor V) and hemin (factor X)
and latex agglutination against PRP.
Meningitis with Hib can be diagnosed
by antigen detection in the cerebrospinal
fluid (CSF).

**What is the *H. influenzae* vaccine
composed of?**

The *H. influenzae* type B (Hib) vaccine is
made of type B capsular polysaccharide
conjugated to a protein (e.g., diphtheria
toxoid) that allows for a T-dependent
immune response providing greater
protection than T-independent immune
response.

**What is the pathognomonic radio-
graphic sign seen with epiglottitis?**

"Thumb sign" seen on lateral cervical x-ray as manifestation of enlarged
epiglottis.

***Haemophilus influenzae* is known for
causing epiglottitis in children. How
does this present?**

An initial sore throat with fever that
progresses to airway obstruction, stridor, dysphagia, and drooling due to an
inability to swallow. The epiglottis is
red and swollen.

**Why has *H. influenzae* remained the
second most common cause of otitis
media in children vaccinated with Hib?**

Ninety percent of otitis media is caused
by a nonencapsulated (nontypeable)
type, thus antibodies against type B are
not protective.

**What diseases are seen in the nonen-
capsulated strains versus encapsulated
type B *H. influenzae*?**

Nonencapsulated (nontypeable) strains
cause local infections such as pneumonia, otitis media, and sinusitis.
Encapsulated strains (usually type B)
cause invasive infections such as meningitis, acute epiglottitis, septic arthritis,
and sepsis.

Why are patients with sickle cell disease especially susceptible to *H. influenzae* infection?

The spleen is necessary to clear encapsulated organisms and sickle cell disease results in functional asplenia.

What are the treatment options for *H. influenzae*?

Local infections are treated with amoxicillin with clavulanate or second- or third-generation cephalosporin. Invasive infections are treated with third-generation cephalosporins such as ceftriaxone that can cross the blood-brain barrier to treat meningitis.

What drug is used for prophylaxis for close contacts?

Rifampin achieves a high concentration in secretions, thereby reducing spread.

BORDETELLA PERTUSSIS

What disease does *Bordetella pertussis* cause?

Pertussis or whooping cough

How is *B. pertussis* diagnosed?

Bacterial culture (on Bordet-Gengou agar) or polymerase chain reaction (PCR) from nasopharyngeal swab or serology

What culture media does *B. pertussis* require for growth?

Bordet-Gengou (potato) agar or Regan-Lowe medium. Note that *B. pertussis* is difficult to culture.

What are the three stages of whooping cough?

1. Catarrhal (1–2 weeks with symptoms similar to a viral upper respiratory infection [URI]; most contagious stage)
2. Paroxysmal (following 1–6 weeks with characteristic burst of cough with inspiratory "whoop")
3. Convalescent (2–3 weeks with decreased coughing attacks; not contagious)

What are the virulence factors of *B. pertussis*?

Attachment virulence factors (filamentous hemagglutinin [FHA]) and toxins (pertussis toxin, tracheal cytotoxin, and invasive adenylate cyclase)

What is the mechanism of action of filamentous hemagglutinin (FHA)?

FHA facilitates attachment to the cilia of respiratory epithelial cells.

What is the mechanism of action of tracheal cytotoxin?

Ciliostasis and epithelial cell death, resulting in diminishing mucociliary clearance

What is the mechanism of action of pertussis toxin?

Pertussis toxin inactivates G_i via adenosine diphosphate (ADP) ribosylation. Inactivated G_i cannot inhibit adenylate cyclase; therefore, there is increased cyclic adenosine monophosphate (cAMP).

What is the clinical significance of increased cAMP?

Impaired cell function (especially neutrophils, macrophages, lymphocytes) and chemotaxis. Impaired chemotaxis leads to lymphocytosis because lymphocytes stay in circulation instead of migrating into lymphoid tissue.

What is the treatment of whooping cough and when should it be given?

Macrolides (e.g., azithromycin) should be given in the prodromal or catarrhal stage to render the patient noninfectious and prevent spread to contacts. However, treatment does not alter the clinical course of the disease in the source patient.

In whom the majority of whooping cough cases occur today?

Classically unimmunized infants younger than 1 year. However, in the last 10 years adolescent and adult infections are more common than infant infections.

What is the clinical case definition of pertussis?

Cough illness lasting 2 weeks without clear cause and one of the following: paroxysms of coughing, inspiratory whoop, or post-tussive emesis

What vaccines are available for *B. pertussis*?

A killed-whole cell vaccine and an acellular vaccine are available for children under 7 years. Two booster vaccines are also available for adolescents and adults.

PSEUDOMONAS AERUGINOSA

What diseases are commonly associated with *Pseudomonas aeruginosa*?

Pneumonia (cystic fibrosis patients, mechanically ventilated patients), otitis externa (elderly diabetics), wound infections (burn patients), urinary tract infections (hospital patients), corneal ulcers (contact lens wearers), sepsis, endocarditis (intravenous [IV] drug users), osteomyelitis (IV drug users), osteochondritis (following penetration injury to foot), ecthyma gangrenosum, and hot tub folliculitis (hot tub user) **Mnemonic:** **O**h **B**oy **P**seudomonas **SEEM**s **U**nhealthy (**O**steomyelitis, **B**urn victims, **P**neumonia, **S**epsis, **E**ndocarditis, **E**cthyma gangrenosum, **M**alignant external otitis, **U**TIs)

Describe the important biochemical characteristics of *P. aeruginosa*:

Obligates aerobe that grows on blood or MacConkey agar; does not ferment lactose (colorless on MacConkey); is oxidase positive; produces pyoverdin (green pigment fluoresces under ultraviolet light); pyocyanin (blue); and polar flagella.

What is the characteristic smell of *P. aeruginosa*?

Grapelike scent (another description is the smell of wet corn tortillas)

How is *P. aeruginosa* differentiated from Enterobacteriaceae?

All will grow on MacConkey agar, but *P. aeruginosa* is oxidase positive and lactose negative.

What is the mechanism of exotoxin A produced by *P. aeruginosa*?

Exotoxin A inhibits elongation factor 2 (EF-2), thereby inhibiting protein synthesis.

Which other toxin producing bacteria also inhibits EF-2?

Corynebacterium diphtheriae

What three groups of patients are extremely susceptible to *P. aeruginosa* infections?

1. Burn patients
2. Cystic fibrosis patients
3. Neutropenic patients

What is a common source of *P. aeruginosa*?

Pseudomonas aeruginosa is a water-loving organism and its common sources include hospital respiratory equipment, sinks, basins, AC units, and plants.

Why is *P. aeruginosa* one of the most feared bacteria?	It is ubiquitous, causes a large variety of diseases, can be very virulent in compromised hosts, and is relatively antibiotic resistant.
What is the clinical significance of ecthyma gangrenosum?	An ulcerated lesion with black eschar. It appears almost exclusively in *Pseudomonas* sepsis (typically in neutropenic patients) and requires immediate medical attention and antibiotic coverage.
What characteristics of *P. aeruginosa* allow it aggressively invade tissues?	Elastases allow *P. aeruginosa* to invade skin creating erythema gangrenosum and progress to sepsis.
What is the treatment of *P. aeruginosa*?	For severe infections, typically a pseudomonas-specific penicillin (ticarcillin, piperacillin) or cephalosporin (ceftazidime, cefepime) plus an aminoglycoside (gentamicin, tobramycin, amikacin; recall excellent for aerobic bacteria) or a pseudomonas-specific fluoroquinolone (ciprofloxacin)

LEGIONELLA PNEUMOPHILA

What diseases does *Legionella pneumophila* cause?	Legionnaires' disease and Pontiac fever
How does Legionnaires' disease present?	Severe atypical lobar pneumonia with neurologic (mental confusion) and gastrointestinal (nonbloody diarrhea) complaints
What is the general demography of individuals presenting with *Legionella*?	Middle-aged and elderly individuals
What are the risk factors for Legionnaires' disease?	Cigarette smoking, alcoholics, chronic lung disease, and immunosuppressed states
Where is *L. pneumophila* found within infected patients? Why?	Intracellularly in alveolar monocytes/macrophages. It is a facultative intracellular organism that inhibits phagosome-lysosome fusion and replicates within the phagosome.

How is Legionnaires' disease diagnosed?

Most commonly with culture on selective media (buffered charcoal yeast extract agar; iron and cysteine are required growth factors) and urinary antigen test

What would be abnormal on a basic metabolic panel in a patient with *L. pneumophila?*

Hyponatremia

What stain is required to visualize *L. pneumophila?*

Silver staining or immunofluorescent staining. *Legionella pneumophila* stains poorly with Gram staining because it is an intracellular pathogen.

What have been the major sources for Legionnaires' disease?

Water sources (air conditioners, water distribution systems, and the like) due to inhalation of aerosolized particles. Person-to-person transmission does not occur.

What are the treatment options for Legionnaires' disease?

Mortality from Legionnaires' disease can approach 30% to 50% in untreated patients, so they need rapid treatment with macrolides (azithromycin, erythromycin), fluoroquinolones, or tetracyclines.

What are the signs and symptoms of Pontiac fever and how does it differ from Legionnaires' disease?

Pontiac fever includes generalized headache, fevers, chills, and myalgias without any respiratory complaints. It is generally a self-limited illness that does not require treatment and resolves within 1 week.

KLEBSIELLA PNEUMONIAE

Describe the biochemical characteristics of *Klebsiella pneumoniae*.

Lactose-fermenting, encapsulated, non-motile (i.e., lacks H antigen)

What diseases are caused by *Klebsiella pneumoniae*?

Necrotizing lobar pneumonia, nosocomial UTIs, bacteremia, and wound infection

Describe the appearance of *K. pneumoniae* colonies and what gives them this appearance:

Appear as *mucoid colonies* due to large capsule size

What population is especially susceptible to *K. pneumoniae* and what is the characteristic appearance of the sputum?	Alcoholics, diabetics, hospitalized patients with "red-currant jelly" sputum
Which antibiotics are used to treat Klebsiella?	First- and second-generation cephalosporins, vancomycin

CLINICAL VIGNETTES

An older man with a significant history of smoking and alcohol consumption presents with a fever, nonproductive cough, and shortness of breath. Several of his coworkers have had similar symptoms over the preceding months, and his workplace is investigating whether the air conditioner may be a source of infection. He also uses a humidifier in his home. What is the likely diagnosis and organism? How is the organism visualized?

Legionella pneumonia (Legionnaires' disease) caused by *L. pneumophila*. Visualize with silver stain or fluorescence staining

A young child presents with a 2-week history of mild upper respiratory symptoms and a severe paroxysmal cough, followed by high-pitched inspiratory *whoop*. A complete blood count (CBC) reveals marked lymphocytosis. What is the likely diagnosis and causative organism?

Whooping cough or pertussis caused by *B. pertussis*

This bacterium, which has reservoirs in water sources, causes *hot tub folliculitis*, characterized by pruritic or tender follicular lesions following bathing in a hot tub, whirlpool, or public swimming pool.

Pseudomonas aeruginosa

A 10-year-old girl with cystic fibrosis presents with 2 days of high fever and a cough productive of purulent green sputum. On chest x-ray (CXR) there is a left upper lobe (LUL) infiltrate. What is the most likely pathogen contributing to her symptoms? Appropriate treatment?

Pseudomonas aeruginosa. Treatment with an aminoglycoside and antipseudomonal penicillin (e.g., tobramycin and piperacillin) or an antipseudomonal cephalosporin

A 70-year-old man with diabetes presents with severe left ear pain and discharge. On physical examination, there is granulation tissue seen in the ear canal.

Pseudomonas is the most common cause of malignant otitis externa.

CHAPTER 11

Gram-Negative Rods (Zoonotic)

Name the five medically important zoonotic gram-negative rods:	1. *Yersinia* 2. *Francisella* 3. *Brucella* 4. *Pasteurella* 5. *Bartonella* **Mnemonic:** Find **Bru**tal **Ba**cteria on **Y**our **P**ets (*Francisella*, **Bru***cella*, **Ba***rtonella*, **Y***ersinia*, **P***asteurella*)
Which zoonotic organisms are facultative intracellular organisms?	*Francisella*, *Brucella*, and *Yersinia*

YERSINIA

Describe the morphology of *Yersinia pestis*:	Nonmotile, bipolar staining pleomorphic gram-negative coccobacillus
What diseases does *Y. pestis* cause?	Bubonic plague (most common), septicemic plague, and pneumonic plague
How is *Y. pestis* typically transmitted?	Rat-flea bite/contact with infected animal (bubonic plague) or via respiratory aerosols (pneumonic plague)
What are the important animal reservoirs for *Y. pestis*?	Rats (worldwide) and prairie dogs (United States)
How virulent is *Y. pestis*?	Extremely. One to ten organisms can cause disease.
Name the important virulence factors for *Y. pestis*:	F1 envelope antigen, V antigen, W antigen, endotoxin

What is the purpose of the F1 envelope antigen?

Inhibits phagocytosis and allows *Y. pestis* to survive intracellularly in the lymph nodes causing necrosis and buboes

What is the progression of disease in a person infected with *Y. pestis*?

Initially lymph nodes will swell and become erythematous, warm, and painful (*buboes*). Then fever and myalgia begin. Next, lung infection (pneumonic plague, virtually fatal) and sepsis may occur.

Why is the bubonic plague referred to as the *Black Death*?

Cutaneous hemorrhage and disseminated intravascular coagulation cause a black skin discoloration.

How is *Y. pestis* infection treated?

Streptomycin, gentamicin, or doxycycline

What type of vaccine against *Y. pestis* is available? What is its limitation?

A killed whole-cell vaccine protects against bubonic plague and not pneumonic plague.

How is *Yersinia enterocolitica* transmitted to humans and what does it cause?

Consumption of contaminated meat, cat and dog feces, and unpasteurized milk leads to enterocolitis (fever and bloody diarrhea), similar to *Salmonella* and *Shigella* infections.

What condition is *Yersinia enterocolitica* infection often confused with?

Appendicitis. *Yersinia enterocolitica* causes mesenteric adenitis (focal ulcerations in the ileum with swelling of the with fever, right lower quadrant pain, and leukocytosis).

How is *Y. enterocolitica* treated?

Treat with either fluoroquinolones or trimethoprim-sulfamethoxazole (TMP- SMX). It is resistant to cephalosporins.

What is the most common postinfectious sequelae?

Erythema nodosum and reactive arthritis (more common in Northern Europe and HLA-B27 tissue type)

FRANCISELLA TULARENSIS

Francisella tularensis **causes two forms of tularemia, describe both forms:**

1. Ulceroglandular form (70%–80%; handling of infected animals) presents with ulcers at the site of infection, lymphadenopathy at the draining lymph nodes, and fever.
2. The more severe typhoidal form (10%–15%; ingestion) often includes pneumonia and symptoms of bacteremia (fevers, chills, myalgias, malaise, and weight loss).

How is *F. tularensis* spread?

Via vectors (wood ticks, deer-flies, mosquitoes) and handling of infected animals (especially rabbits and deer). In the United States, it is most commonly acquired from ticks. Hunters often acquire the pneumonic form of the infection due to aerosolization of the pathogen during skinning of animals.

How virulent is *F. tularensis*?

Highly virulent. Requires only 10 to 50 organisms to cause disease. Most diagnostic laboratories will not culture it, and there is concern over its use as a bioterrorism agent.

What special culture requirement does *Francisella tularensis* have?

Most strains require cysteine.

What is required for host defense against *F. tularensis*?

Cell-mediated immunity as *F. tularensis* is an intracellular pathogen.

How is *F. tularensis* diagnosed?

Serological tests since laboratory culture is dangerous

What is the drug of choice for the treatment of *F. tularensis*?

Streptomycin

BRUCELLA

What type of cells does *Brucella* infect?	Reticuloendothelial system (lymph nodes, spleen, liver, and bone marrow)
What is the most characteristic symptom of brucellosis?	Undulant (a diurnal rising and falling) fever actually occurs in a minority of patients. Fever is normal in the morning, has slow rise throughout day, and peaks in the PM. Most patients have nonspecific symptoms (fever, malaise), myalgias, lymphadenitis hepatosplenomegaly, and pancytopenia. The presentation may also be dominated by chronic pain in affected tissues such as the spine.
Who is most likely to acquire brucellosis?	Those with close contact with livestock (farmers, veterinarians, meat packers) and those who drink unpasteurized milk
What is the treatment of choice for Brucella?	Doxycycline plus rifampin or doxycycline plus streptomycin

PASTEURELLA MULTOCIDA

What is the typical source of *Pasteurella multocida* in human infections?	Cat or dog bites (their normal oral flora) or cat scratch
How does *P. multocida* most commonly present?	Painful wound infection with rapid swelling within 24 hours of bite
Why shouldn't wounds from animal bites be sutured up?	*Pasteurella multocida* is a facultative anaerobe and suturing the wound would provide a better growth environment for the bacteria.
What drugs are used as treatment and prophylaxis for *P. multocida*?	Treat with penicillin G and prophylaxis with amoxicillin/clavulanate. *Pasteurella multocida* is resistant to first-generation cephalosporins.

BARTONELLA

What diseases does *Bartonella henselae* cause?	Cat scratch disease and bacillary angiomatosis
What is cat scratch disease? What patient population is most often affected?	Cutaneous lesion at the site of cat scratch/bite with regional lymphadenopathy, fever, and malaise. Eighty-five to ninety percent of cases occur in children.
What is seen on a lymph node biopsy of cat scratch disease?	Stellate granulomas
What stain may be used on histopathologic examination to strongly suggest cat scratch disease?	Warthin-Starry stain
What is the treatment of cat scratch disease?	Azithromycin, quinolones, or doxycycline. More serious infections need combined therapy with rifampin.
What is bacillary angiomatosis? What patient population is affected?	Systemic disease often presents with cutaneous vascular lesions that easily bleed in AIDS patients (can therefore be consumed with Kaposi sarcoma).
What is the treatment of bacillary angiomatosis?	Oral erythromycin or doxycycline. Newer macrolides such as azithromycin and clarithromycin probably effective but not as well studied
What diseases does *Bartonella quintana* cause?	Trench fever, bacillary angiomatosis (several species of *Bartonella* are known to cause bacillary angiomatosis) and endocarditis in homeless patients
What is trench fever?	Disease that affected up to 1 million soldiers during World War I. Typically presents with flu-like illness with bone pain, splenomegaly, and a maculopapular rash. It is spread by human body louse.
What stain can be used to visualize Bartonella species?	Warthin Starry stain
What does Coxeilla burnetti cause?	Q fever

CLINICAL VIGNETTES

A patient of yours kills a deer infected with F. tularensis; he then skins it. His wife then prepares the deer for dinner but undercooks it. The deer is served at her office for lunch the next day. What type of infection will the husband present with? What type will his wife and her coworkers present with?

> Hunter: pneumonia through inhalation of aerosolized bacteria from skinning or ulceroglandular from inoculation. Wife and coworkers: typhoidal tularemia with fever and abdominal pain

A 25-year-old woman presents with a painful rash on her hand and tender axillary adenopathy for 2 days. She owns two cats. On examination, she has multiple pruritic erythematous vesicles and papules on her right hand with suppurative axillary adenopathy. What is the diagnosis? Treatment?

> Cat scratch disease. Azithromycin

A 5-year-old girl presents to the emergency department (ED) with a deep puncture wound on her hand from a cat bite. There is considerable pain, erythema, and swelling noted. What is required for prophylaxis?

> Amox-clavulanate for *Pasteurella* prophylaxis

A 30-year-old human immunodeficiency virus (HIV)-positive man presents with 1 week of fever and malaise. On his forearm there is a 2-cm round, vascular, nontender, friable exophytic lesion. He recently returned from a trip to South America. He lives at home alone with two dogs and 2 cats. What is the diagnosis? Pathogen? Appropriate treatment?

> Bacillary angiomatosis caused by *Bartonella*. Oral erythromycin, doxycycline, or azithromycin

CHAPTER 12

Mycobacteria (Tuberculosis, Leprosy)

What are some characteristics of mycobacteria?	Obligate aerobes, acid-fast bacilli, intracellular growth, and multiple-drug resistance
How are mycobacteria visualized under light microscope?	Appear red with Ziehl-Neelsen acid-fast stain. Stain is positive for AFB = "acid-fast bacillus" Tuberculosis (TB) stain poorly with Gram stain; technically gram positive but not useful in clinical practice
What is the principal dye in acid-fast stain and what component of the cell wall does it bind?	Carbolfuchsin binds to mycolic acid (long- chain fatty acid), which is present in abundance in the cell wall.
What other bacteria are acid-fast? Why?	*Nocardia* species are acid-fast because their cell walls are also high in mycolic acid.
What two classic "ancient" diseases are caused by mycobacteria?	Tuberculosis ("consumption") by *Mycobacterium tuberculosis* and leprosy (Hansen disease) by *Mycobacterium leprae*

MYCOBACTERIUM TUBERCULOSIS

What populations are most at risk for TB?	Elderly persons, immunocompromised, human immunodeficiency virus (HIV)/ immunosuppressed (transplant patients), incarcerated populations, and people from lower socioeconomic status
What is the main host defense against *M. tuberculosis*?	Cell-mediated immunity (CD4$^+$ T cells and macrophages)

Purified protein derivative (PPD) is a skin test for tuberculosis. How does it work?

Intradermally injected proteins from *M. tuberculosis* initiate a local delayed-type hypersensitivity reaction (type IV hyper- sensitivity) in previously infected individuals.

What are the criteria for a positive PPD skin test?

A positive test is defined based on the size of the red, raised induration after 48 hours: greater than 15 mm for persons with no known exposure, greater than 10 mm in high-risk patients (including health-care workers), greater than 5 mm in HIV patients or those with recent known exposure

How is latent tuberculosis (TB) infection detected and how is it treated?

Latent infection is conversion to positive PPD with no signs or symptoms of active disease and no signs of disease on chest x-ray (CXR). First-line treatment is 9 months of isoniazid.

What medication must be coadministered to all patients on isoniazid therapy and why?

Vitamin B_6 (pyridoxine) to prevent a peripheral neuropathy

What can cause a false-positive PPD?

Bacillus Calmette-Guérin (BCG) vaccine, prior treated tuberculosis (once exposed, the PPD remains positive even after treatment), exposure to nontuberculosis mycobacteria

How is *M. tuberculosis* cultured?

Lowenstein-Jensen agar. However, it is important to remember that TB is very difficult to culture and takes weeks to grow.

How is tuberculosis transmitted?

Inhalation of infected respiratory droplets

What is primary tuberculosis?

An infection in the lungs of a previously unexposed individual. Normally seen in the middle or lower lobes of the lungs.

Pathology Correlate: Describe the pathogenesis of primary tuberculosis:

Mycobacteria ingested by phagocytes trigger cell-mediated immunity leading to caseating granulomas.

What are the clinical manifestations of most primary infections with tuberculosis?

No symptoms (asymptomatic 90%), positive PPD, Ghon complex

What groups are at risk for symptomatic primary tuberculosis?

Those with deficient cell-mediated immunity (children, elderly, immunocompromised, or immunosuppressed)

Pathology correlate: What is the pathology of symptomatic primary tuberculosis?

In the lungs and other organs, large caseous granulomas develop and eventually liquefy, creating cavitary lesions with air-fluid levels (air-fluid levels in the lungs only).

Pathology correlate: The Ghon complex is the hallmark of primary tuberculosis, what is it?

Ghon complex = a Ghon focus (calcified TB granuloma forming a nodule in the middle or lower lung) + an associated hilar or perihilar lymph node

What is secondary tuberculosis?

Reactivation of a prior infection due to weakened immunity (months to years later). Most adult cases of active tuberculosis are secondary tuberculosis. Normally seen in the apical lungs.

What are the signs and symptoms of active pulmonary tuberculosis?

Cough with hemoptysis, low-grade fever, night sweats, and weight loss. Chest radiograph showing hilar adenopathy, upper lobe infiltrates (due to higher oxygen saturation), cavitary lesions

What is the treatment of active tuberculosis?

Cough with hemoptysis, low-grade 6-month regimen: initially four drugs (rifampin, isoniazid, pyrazinamide, ethambutol) for 2 months, followed by 4 months of isoniazid and rifampin. Multiple drugs should always be used to prevent the emergence of multidrug-resistant strains.

What are the main toxicities of anti-tuberculous therapy?

Rifampin → orange discoloration of urine/tears, hepatitis, drug interactions Isoniazid → hepatitis, peripheral neuropathy, lupus-like syndrome Pyrazinamide → hepatitis, hyperuricemia Ethambutol → optic neuritis Streptomycin → nephro- and ototoxicity

What should be supplemented with isoniazid therapy?

Pyrodoxine/B6. To prevent peripheral neuropathy

What percentage of primary infections progress to active tuberculosis?

Five percent of those primarily infected will develop reactivation tuberculosis in the first 1 to 2 years. Another 5% will develop reactivation infection sometime later in life. Normal infected individuals have a 10% lifetime risk of active infection, while immunocompromised patients are at substantially higher risk.

What is miliary tuberculosis?

Disseminated TB infection leading to millet seed-sized granulomas in the lungs, liver, spleen, bone, kidneys, spine, and other organs

Who gets miliary tuberculosis?

Those with weakened cell-mediated immunity (HIV positive, elderly, children)

What is Pott disease?

Tuberculous infection of the thoracic/lumbar spine leading to destruction of intervertebral discs/bodies and compression fractures

What is the most common extrapulmonary manifestation of tuberculosis?

Scrofula or cervical mycobacterial lymphadenitis

What is the most common cause of adrenal insufficiency worldwide?

Adrenal TB

MYCOBACTERIUM LEPRAE

What are the two main clinical manifestations of leprosy?

1. Lepromatous leprosy
2. Tuberculoid leprosy

What is lepromatous leprosy?

Malignant, progressive form of leprosy that results from failure of Th-2 cell-mediated immunity and primarily affects the nerves, skin, eyes, and testes, leading to loss of sensation in symmetric stocking-glove distribution, leonine facies (thickened facial skin), nodular skin lesions, saddle-nose deformity, blindness, and infertility. Sensory loss can lead to repetitive trauma and secondary infection, eventually leading to loss of fingers and toes. In lepromatous leprosy biopsies of lesions may show large numbers of organisms and minimal host inflammatory response.

What is tuberculoid leprosy?

Benign form of leprosy that is mild and sometimes self-limiting disease in a person with intact cell-mediated immunity. Usually only one or two hypopigmented, hairless macular skin lesions with diminished sensation. Enlarged nerves near the skin may be palpable (greater auricular, ulnar, posterior tibial, peroneal). In contrast to lepromatous leprosy, there is usually asymmetric nerve involvement. In tuberculoid leprosy biopsies of lesions may show small numbers of organisms and vigorous granuloma formation.

What laboratory test distinguishes between lepromatous and tuberculoid leprosies?

Lepromin skin test is negative in lepromatous leprosy. Positive in tuberculoid leprosy

How is leprosy transmitted?

Respiratory secretions or contact with skin lesions of infected individual. However, not all individuals are susceptible to infection (reasons unknown).

What conditions favor the growth of *M. leprae*?

Low temperature (30°C). *Mycobacterium leprae* preferentially affects cool areas of the body (surface of the skin in distal extremities and the nose).

How is *M. leprae* cultured or grown?

Mycobacterium leprae cannot be cultured on artificial media, and has been grown on mouse footpads and in armadillos (doubling time of 14 days).

What is the main host defense against leprosy?

Cell-mediated immunity (CD4$^+$ T cells and macrophages) because *M. leprae* is a facultative intracellular pathogen

What is the treatment of leprosy?

Dapsone and rifampin for tuberculoid form. Add clofazimine for lepromatous form. Because of slow growth rate, must treat for at least 2 years

What are potential toxicities associated with dapsone treatment?

Methemoglobinemia and hemolysis

How are close contacts prophylactically treated?

Dapsone

ATYPICAL MYCOBACTERIA

What is *Mycobacterium avium* complex (MAC) and what are its symptoms?

A mycobacterium ubiquitous in water and soil, but has become a common pathogen in late-stage AIDS patients (CD4 count <50). Symptoms include chronic wasting, fever, weight loss, marrow suppression, and chronic watery diarrhea. May also cause respiratory disease mimicking tuberculosis especially in chronic obstructive pulmonary disease (COPD) patients.

What causes *fish-tank* or *swimming-pool* granuloma?

Mycobacterium marinum. Granulomatous, ulcerating lesions at the site of breaks in the skin exposed to these environments

CLINICAL VIGNETTES

A 22-year-old woman is taking isoniazid prophylaxis for tuberculosis exposure. After 1 month of therapy she develops tingling in both her hands. What is the term for what she is experiencing and how would you treat her?

Peripheral neuropathy due to vitamin B_6 depletion by the isoniazid (INH). Treat with vitamin B_6, otherwise known as pyridoxine

A patient presents with low-grade fever, chills, night sweats, weight loss, and a cough productive of blood-tinged sputum for 2 months. You suspect tuberculosis (TB) and order a chest x-ray. What findings on chest x-ray would be consistent with your suspected diagnosis?

Active tuberculosis pneumonia with cavitary lesions and posterior upper lobe involvement (past exposure would show isolated granuloma, Ghon focus, Ghon complex, old scarring in the upper lobes)

A 34-year-old male immigrant presents to the physician with a cough and fever. On his last visit 12 months ago, his PPD was positive and chest x-ray showed likely active tuberculosis. He was treated with INH and rifampin and his symptoms abated. On this visit, he appears very sick and has hard time breathing. He denies night sweats and hemoptysis. His temperature is 102.1°F. Chest x-ray reveals infiltrates in the right middle and lower lobes and a Ghon complex. He is still taking INH and rifampin, which do not seem to help. What is the most likely diagnosis?

TB relapse; note that the Ghon complex is consistent with primary healed TB and does not exclude reactivation on relapse.

A 30-year-old woman from Southeast Asia presents with a hypopigmented, macular forearm lesion and associated with loss of sensation (decreased pin prick). The arm shows significant muscle atrophy. What is the most likely diagnosis?

Tuberculoid leprosy

CHAPTER 13

Actinomyces, Nocardia, Mycoplasma

ACTINOMYCES ISRAELII

Describe the appearance of *Actinomyces israelii* on light microscopy:

Gram-positive rods forming branching, beaded filaments. Colonies in pus appear as yellow granules called *sulfur granules*.

Where is *Actinomyces* normally found?

In the gingival crevices of the teeth, especially in patients with poor oral hygiene. It forms part of the normal oral flora.

What are *sulfur* granules of *Actinomyces*?

Yellow-colored colonies and cellular debris (do not actually contain sulfur) that are visible within the purulent discharge

Can *Actinomyces* grow without oxygen?

Yes. *Actinomyces* is an anaerobe.

How does an *Actinomyces* infection manifest?

Actinomyces causes eroding abscesses with draining sinus tracts. Main forms are cervicofacial (*lumpy jaw*) and thoracic. Also may cause pelvic pathology in females.

How are *Actinomyces* infections treated?

Penicillin G (often for a prolonged course) +/− surgical drainage

NOCARDIA ASTEROIDES

Describe the appearance of *Nocardia asteroides* on light microscopy:	Gram-positive rods forming branching, beaded filaments. *Nocardia* is also slightly acid-fast due to the mycolic acid in its cell walls. It is also catalase positive.
Where is *Nocardia* normally found?	In the soil with transmission via inhalation. *Nocardia* is never a normal flora.
Does *Nocardia* require oxygen?	Yes. *Nocardia* is aerobic, in contrast to Actinomyces, an anaerobe.
How is *Nocardia* transmitted?	Transmitted via inhalation, producing lung abscesses and cavitations (it can be confused with *Mycobacterium tuberculosis*)
How does a *Nocardia* infection manifest?	Infection with *Nocardia* can produce pneumonia, lung abscesses, and can spread systemically. Abscesses can form throughout the body, especially in the brain. Commonly described as "cavitary lesions."
What risk factors predispose to *Nocardia* infection?	Immunosuppression and cancer
How is nocardiosis treated?	Trimethoprim-sulfamethoxazole (TMP-SMX) Mneumonic: SNAP (Sulfonamide Nocardia, Actinomyces Penicillin)

MYCOPLASMA

Why do penicillins and cephalosporins not work against *Mycoplasma*?	*Mycoplasma* has no cell wall; therefore, penicillins and cephalosporins that target the cell wall are ineffective.
What component of *Mycoplasma* cell membrane is unique?	It contains sterols like cholesterol and is the cell's only protective layer. *Mycoplasma* requires cholesterol for growth.
What is unique about the size of *Mycoplasma*?	They are the smallest free-living organisms capable of self-replication.

Name two *Mycoplasma* species that cause disease in humans:	1. *Mycoplasma* pneumoniae (Eaton agent) 2. *Ureaplasma urealyticum*
In what population is *Mycoplasma pneumoniae* the most common cause of pneumonia?	"Walking pneumonia" in teenagers and young adults
What is "walking pneumonia"?	A community-acquired pneumonia usually caused by *M. pneumoniae* in which the radiologic findings appear much worse than the patient's symptoms
How is *M. pneumoniae* transmitted?	Inhalation of respiratory droplets
Name a laboratory test for *M. pneumoniae*:	Infection leads to production of antibodies against *M. pneumoniae* antigens, resulting in a positive cold agglutinin test.
How can *M. pneumoniae* be cultured?	On Eaton agar
What is the prognosis of *M. pneumoniae* pneumonia and how is it treated?	Pneumonia is self-limiting, but macrolides or tetracyclines can shorten the course.
Where is *U. urealyticum* normally found?	In the normal flora of the lower urinary tract of 60% of sexually active women
What infection is caused by *Ureaplasma* and how is it treated?	Urethritis with dysuria and clear mucoid discharge. Treat with tetracycline macrolide or a tetracycline.
How can *Ureaplasma* urethritis be distinguished from other causes of urethritis (e.g., *Neisseria*, *Chlamydia*)?	*Ureaplasma* has urease, and can split urea to ammonia and CO_2.

CLINICAL VIGNETTES

A 47-year-old male patient was found to have an oral abscess that drains through a sinus tract in the skin. When the organism was cultured, it produced yellow granules. What is the organism and what is the treatment of choice?

Actinomyces israelii, penicillin

A 50-year-old alcoholic with poor dentition comes in with 1 week of chest wall pain, fevers, and chills. A lesion from the left side of his chest is draining serosanguinous fluid and laboratory analysis shows a gram-positive branching rod. What is the most likely diagnosis? What is the appropriate antibiotic therapy?

Actinomyces, penicillin

A human immunodeficiency virus (HIV)-positive patient with a CD4 count of 100 was found to have a brain abscess that contained a gram-positive organism that stains weakly acid-fast. What is the organism and what is the treatment for choice?

Nocardia asteroides, trimethoprim-sulfamethoxazole (TMP-SMX)

A 29-year-old liver transplant patient presents with fever, anorexia, night sweats, weight loss, and a productive cough for 1 week. His purified protein derivative (PPD) is 3 mm and his chest x-ray (CXR) shows a right upper lobe cavitation. Sputum examination shows acid-fast branching rods. What is the most likely diagnosis?

Nocardia. Remember to keep *Nocardia* in the differential for a cavitary lung lesion in an immunocompromised patient.

CHAPTER 14

Spirochetes

What are the main classes of spirochetes?	**Mnemonic:** *Borrelia, Leptospira, Treponema* **BLT**
How do you visualize spirochetes?	On dark-field microscopy

TREPONEMA PALLIDUM

What disease does *Treponema pallidum* cause?	Syphilis
How is syphilis transmitted?	Sexually or transplacentally
What are the stages of syphilis?	Primary (3–6 weeks after initial infection), secondary (~6 weeks after resolution of primary chancre), latent (after resolution of secondary), tertiary (6–40 years after infection)
How does primary syphilis manifest?	A painless chancre on the genitalia or perianal region that may be accompanied by nontender swelling of regional inguinal lymph nodes (groin adenitis)
Describe the chancre of primary syphilis:	Ulcerating, painless lesion that is highly infectious
Describe the symptoms of secondary syphilis:	The bacteremic/disseminated stage with systemic symptoms (fever, weight loss, etc), a classic maculopapular rash often involving the palms and soles, and condyloma latum (warty lesion) in warm moist areas (groin, skin folds)
What is latent syphilis?	Latent syphilis occurs after secondary syphilis has resolved. All patients are asymptomatic with a positive blood test for syphilis without any signs or symptoms of disease.

What is the natural history of latent syphilis?

In the first 2 years (early latent), 25% may relapse to secondary syphilis. Over many years, 30% may progress to tertiary syphilis.

What are the main categories of tertiary syphilis?

Gummatous syphilis, cardiovascular syphilis, and neurosyphilis

When does tertiary syphilis develop? What are gummas?

After 6 to 40 years soft, noncancerous granulomatous growths of tertiary syphilis

How does cardiovascular syphilis manifest?

Classically a thoracic aneurysm forms in the *ascending* aorta or aortic arch leading to aortic insufficiency or dissection.

What are the manifestations of neurosyphilis?

Aseptic meningitis (predominantly lymphocytes in cerebrospinal fluid [CSF]), meningovascular syphilis (vascular damage leading to cerebrovascular occlusion or infarction), tabes dorsalis, and general paresis

When should you suspect neurosyphilis as the cause of a stroke?

Stroke without hypertension in an individual with a history of sexually transmitted diseases (STDs)

What is tabes dorsalis?

Syphilitic damage to the *posterior columns* and dorsal roots of the spinal cord with impairment of position and vibration sense. May result in broad-based gait ataxia and a positive Romberg test

What is general paresis?

A form of neurosyphilis presenting with insidious psychiatric symptoms (irritability, apathy) and progressing to a severe dementia

What is Argyll-Robertson pupil?

A feature of tertiary syphilis, it is a pupil that constricts during accommodation but not in response to light (i.e., *prostitute's pupil "accommodates but doesn't react"*)

Mnemonic: GeT A SCAR w/Treponema (**G**ummas, **T**abes dorsalis, **A**ortic aneurysm, **S**yphilis, **C**hancre, **A**rgyll Robinson, **R**ash)

What are the classic findings of congenital syphilis?

Snuffles (bloody nasal discharge), saddle nose, saber shins (bowing of the tibia), Hutchinson teeth (widely spaced, notched upper incisors), rash, neurosyphilis with eighth nerve deafness

Mnemonic: SyphiliS RASH (Snuffles, Saddle nose, Rash, Auditory [deafness], Saber shins, Hutchinson teeth)

What is the treatment of syphilis?

Penicillin (The particular type and dosing of the penicillin depends on the stage of the disease.). Tetracyclines, ceftriaxone, and azithromycin for penicillin-allergic.

What serologic tests are used to screen for syphilis?

Venereal Disease Research Laboratory (VDRL), rapid plasma reagin (RPR), the fluorescent treponemal antibody-absorbed (FTA-ABS), and the Microhemagglutination Assay-Treponema Pallidum (MHA-TP)

Which serologic tests are specific for antibodies against _T. pallidum_ and which are not? Which ones become negative with treatment?

Specific: FTA-ABS and MHA-TP test for antibodies against _T. pallidum_. These are the first serologic tests to become positive and remain positive after treatment.
Nonspecific: VDRL and RPR tests for antibodies are associated with the infection and become negative with treatment.

Describe VDRL and RPR in terms of sensitivity and specificity for syphilis:

VDRL and RPR are highly sensitive but have low specificity.

What may cause a false-positive VDRL?

Viral infections (Epstein-Barr virus [EBV], hepatitides), Drugs, pregnancy, Rheumatic fever, Rheumatoid arthritis, Lupus, and Leprosy

What is a Jarisch-Herxheimer reaction?

Fever, malaise/headache, and myalgias that can occur at the onset of syphilis treatment due to pyrogens released from killed organisms

What is another disease caused by another specifies of _Treponema_?

Treponema pertenue causes yaws.

What are the clinical manifestations of the three stages of yaws?	1. Primary: a painless papule develops into a yaw (a large wart-like lesion) 2. Secondary: disseminated yaws of varying appearance that frequently ulcerate and may involve palms and soles 3. Tertiary: widespread bone and soft tissue destruction

BORRELIA BURGDORFERI

What disease does *Borrelia burgdorferi* cause?	Lyme disease
How is *B. burgdorferi* visualized?	*Borrelia burgdorferi* is seen by light microscope with Giemsa or Wright stains. *Borrelia* are much bigger than other spirochetes and do not require dark-field microscopy. **Mnemonic:** *Borrelia* are **Big**
How is Lyme disease transmitted?	By insect vector, the *Ixodes* tick, from a small mammals and birds reservoir
Where is Lyme disease endemic?	In the northeastern, midwestern, and northwestern United States (also endemic in Europe and Asia). Named after Lyme, Connecticut, where it was first reported
During what time of year is Lyme disease most common?	Summer
What are the stages of Lyme disease?	Like syphilis, there are three stages: 1. Primary localized stage (erythemamigrans) 2. Disseminated stage 3. Late chronic stage
What are the manifestations of primary Lyme disease?	Erythema migrans (EM) and nonspecific flu-like symptoms
What is erythema migrans (EM)?	A red, circular, macular rash that spreads with a red advancing border and a clear central region, giving a bull's-eye or target appearance

What are the manifestations of disseminated (stage 2) Lyme disease?	Systemic: fever, malaise Neurologic: aseptic meningitis, Bell palsy, peripheral neuropathy Cardiac: transient AV block, myocarditis Large joints: brief attacks of migratory arthritis (e.g., the knee) Dermatologic: multiple disseminated EM lesions
What are the chronic manifestations of Lyme disease?	Encephalopathy (impaired memory, somnolence) and migratory autoimmune arthritis
How is Lyme disease treated?	If early localized infection, doxycycline, amoxicillin (for children <8 for whom Doxy is contraindicated). If systemic/disseminated, third-generation cephalosporin **Mnemonic: GEt a BAD LIMP W/** Borrelia (**G**iemsa stain, **E**M, **B**ell palsy, **A**V block, **D**oxycycline, **L**yme disease, **I**xodes, **M**igratory arthritis/Meningitis, **P**enicillin, **W**right stain)

BORRELIA RECURRENTIS

What disease does *Borrelia recurrentis* cause?	Relapsing fever
What are the symptoms of relapsing fever?	3- to 6-day episodes of high fever, headaches, myalgias, followed by approximately eight afebrile days, and then 3- to 6-day relapses of fever. Relapses progressively shorten with longer afebrile periods.
How is relapsing fever treated?	IV beta-lactam (penicillin or ceftriaxone)
Why does relapsing fever relapse?	Antigenic variation: *B. recurrentis* changes its surface proteins to evade the immune system.

LEPTOSPIRA INTERROGANS

What are the symptoms of each phase of leptospirosis?	First (leptospiremic) phase: high spiking temperatures, conjunctivitis, headache, and severe muscle aches
	Second (immune) phase: recurrence of leptospiremic symptoms with meningismus
What is Weil disease?	Severe leptospirosis with renal failure, hepatitis, jaundice, mental status changes, and multiorgan hemorrhage
	Mnemonic: Organs in alphabetical order **KLM** (**K**idneys, **L**iver, **M**ind)
How is *Leptospira* transmitted?	Water contaminated with infected urine of dogs, rats, livestock, and wild animals
What is the treatment of *Leptospira*?	Penicillin or doxycycline

CLINICAL VIGNETTES

A 26-year-old urban man presents to you with a painless chancre on his penis. What is the drug of choice for treatment of his disease?

Treponema pallidum is still exquisitely sensitive to benzathine penicillin (penicillin G).

A 35-year-old man presents with impaired proprioception and locomotor ataxia. He has a history of unprotected intercourse with multiple partners. His symptoms are most likely caused by an untreated infection by what organism?

The patient has tertiary syphilis with injury to the dorsal columns of the spinal cord caused by *T. pallidum*.

An 18-year-old woman presents with 2 days of inability to close her right eye. She has a low-grade fever and rash. One month ago she went camping but has no memory of a tick bite. On examination, she has multiple erythematous skin lesions with central clearing and right-sided facial nerve palsy. What is the most likely diagnosis? Most appropriate treatment?

Lyme disease caused by *B. burgdorferi*. Treat with doxycycline.

CHAPTER 15

Chlamydia, Rickettsia, & Miscellaneous Obligate Intracellular Organisms

Which bacteria are obligate intracellular parasites?

Chlamydia and *Rickettsia*

How are these bacteria cultured?

In living cells. *Rickettsia* and *Chlamydia* cannot be cultured on nonliving media because they need to steal adenosine triphosphate (ATP) from living cells to survive.

Mnemonic: Rob Cells of ATP (*Rickettsia, Chlamydia*)

CHLAMYDIA

During its life cycle, *Chlamydia* exists in two forms, the elementary and reticulate bodies. Which one is the extracellular, infectious body and which one is the intracellular, dividing body?

Elementary body is extracellular and infectious
Reticulate body is intracellular and dividing (replicating)

What is unusual about *Chlamydia*'s cell wall? How does this influence choice of antimicrobial therapy?

It lacks muramic acid; therefore, all β-lactam antibiotics are ineffective against *Chlamydia*.

How is *Chlamydia* diagnosed in the laboratory?

Basophilic intracytoplasmic inclusion bodies within epithelial cells are visualized with Giemsa stain or fluorescent antibodies. Also with PCR and serology

Can *Chlamydia* be visualized with Gram stain?

Chlamydia Gram stains quite poorly because it is an intracellular pathogen.

What disease is caused by *Chlamydia trachomatis* serotypes A, B, C?

Trachoma, a chronic conjunctivitis that can lead to corneal scarring (most common cause of preventable blindness worldwide)

Serotypes D-K?

Nongonococcal urethritis (men) and cervicitis/PID (women), both sexually transmitted. Inclusion conjunctivitis (newborns) and infant pneumonia, both transmitted during delivery through infected birth canals

Serotypes L1, L2, L3?

Lymphogranuloma venereum (LGV)
Mnemonic: L for **L**ymphogranuloma

Is there lifelong immunity to *Chlamydia*?

Because of the existence of multiple serotypes, there is no lifelong immunity to *Chlamydia* as reinfection with another serotype is a frequent occurrence.

What are the most common bacterial sexually transmitted diseases?

Urethritis and cervicitis caused by *C. trachomatis*, majority of women infected are asymptomatic

What is pelvic inflammatory disease?

A sequela of cervicitis due to *C. trachomatis* (or *Neisseria gonorrhoeae*) infection. Spread of the infection to the fallopian tubes and ovaries leads to fallopian tube scarring, and risk of infertility and ectopic pregnancy.

What is Fitz-Hugh Curtis Syndrome?

Perihepatitis in the setting of pelvic inflammatory disease typically presents with pleuritic right upper quadrant pain. Commonly associated with Gonorrhea infections.

What type of arthritis is associated with *Chlamydia*?

Reactive arthritis: Triad of arthritis, dysuria, and eye inflammation (Can't see, can't pee, can't climb a tree)

What are the clinical manifestations of lymphogranuloma venereum (LGV)?

Primary: painless, self-limited genital ulcer
Secondary: acute inguinal adenitis (buboes) due to lymphatic spread of infection
Chronic disease may develop resulting in further ulceration, proctocolitis, rectal strictures, rectovaginal fistulas, and elephantiasis.

How is LGV diagnosed?	Serology and PCR. In the past, a skin test using antigen, prepared from *Chlamydia* and known as the Frei test, was used.
What disease is caused by *Chlamydia psittaci*?	Psittacosis, an atypical pneumonia occurring after exposure to infected birds
What disease is caused by *Chlamydia pneumoniae*?	Atypical pneumonia (gradual onset of fever and nonproductive cough, eosinophilia, history of conjunctivitis)
What vascular changes may *Chlamydia pneumoniae* elicit?	Intimal changes with deposition of lipid-laden macrophages, resulting in a fatty streak. Note that the significance of *C. pneumonia* in the pathogenesis of atherosclerosis remains unclear.
How are *C. pneumoniae* and *C. psittaci* transmitted?	Aerosol transmission
How are *Chlamydia* infections treated?	Tetracycline, doxycycline, erythromycin, azithromycin, or a fluoroquinolone
What is the appropriate therapy for chlamydial neonatal conjunctivitis?	Erythromycin eye drops

RICKETTSIA & OTHER OBLIGATE INTRACELLULAR ORGANISMS

How are rickettsiae transmitted?	Through arthropod vectors
What symptoms are associated with most rickettsial infections?	Rash (vasculitis), high fever, severe headache
What is the Weil-Felix reaction?	A test for antibodies to *Proteus vulgaris* antigens used to diagnose rickettsial infection based on the coincidental cross-reactivity with *Rickettsia* (except *C. burnetii*)
What is Rocky Mountain spotted fever (RMSF)?	Fever, headache, conjunctival redness, and petechial rash on palms and soles due to *Rickettsia rickettsii*. RMSF is transmitted by wood tick bites and is actually more common in the southeastern and south central United States.

Where does the rash related to RMSF start? Where does it spread to?	On the ankles and wrists and palms and soles and then spreads to the trunk, and face (centripetal spread)
What is epidemic typhus, and how is it spread?	Fever, headache, rash due to *Rickettsia prowazekii*. Transmitted at times of over-crowding (poverty, war) by human body lice. Characteristic rash consists of pink macules; starts centrally and spreads outward sparing the palms and soles.
What is endemic typhus, and how is it spread?	Fever, headache, rash from *Rickettsia typhi* (less severe than epidemic typhus) spread by rodent-fleas from a rodent reservoir. Note that it is found in urban areas in the United States.
What causes rickettsial pox?	*Rickettsia akari* carried by mites that causes an initial red papule at the bite site, and eventually chickenpox-like vesicles over the body.
What class of antibiotic can be used for all rickettsial infections?	Tetracyclines (e.g., doxycycline)
What disease does *Coxiella burnetii* cause? How does *C. burnetii* spread?	Q fever. Spreads by inhalation of endospores from *placental* products of animals. It is also potential agent of bioterrorism
What are the symptoms of Q fever?	Self-limited flu-like illness, soaking sweats, pneumonia, and can cause hepatitis and endocarditis. Note that there is no rash
How does *C. burnetii* differ from other rickettsiae?	It is transmitted by aerosols rather than an arthropod vector, is not associated with a rash, and has a negative Weil-Felix reaction.

CLINICAL VIGNETTES

A 24-year-old sexually active man presents with dysuria and urethral discharge. Gram stain of the discharge reveals neutrophils but no gram-negative diplococci. What is the diagnosis and treatment?

Most likely nongonococcal urethritis caused by *C. trachomatis* serotypes D-K. However, must treat for all likely causes of urethritis—either doxycycline or azithromycin for *C. trachomatis* and *Ureaplasma urealyticum*, and ceftriaxone for *N. gonorrhoeae*.

A 29-year-old woman and her husband seek your consultation for an inability to conceive. After a thorough workup, you believe the cause to be an undiagnosed infection in the woman. Examination reveals mild cervical motion tenderness; Gram stain of cervical secretions shows neutrophils but no organisms. The inability of the causal bacteria to produce what substance causes it to be an obligate intracellular parasite?

The patient here has pelvic inflammatory disease (PID). The causal organism is *C. trachomatis*, an intracellular parasite that is unable to make adenosine triphosphate (ATP). PID includes endometritis, salpingitis, tubo-ovarian abscess, and pelvic peritonitis. PID increases the risk of infertility as well as ectopic pregnancies.

A 19-year-old man who recently went camping in the northeast United States presents to the student health clinic at his college with fever, headache, and a rash around both his ankles and wrists. What is the most likely pathogen, how is it transmitted, and what would the treatment of choice be?

Rickettsia rickettsii, tick bite, doxycycline

A 1-month-old infant, whose mother has a history of *C. trachomatis* genital infections, develops pneumonitis. How would you confirm the diagnosis of chlamydial pneumonitis?

Exudates from the respiratory tract revealing cytoplasmic inclusions in epithelial cells seen with Giemsa stain or by immunofluorescence, cell culture treated with cycloheximide, and serologic tests

A young man presents with enlarged tender inguinal lymph nodes with draining sinuses and painful genital ulcers. He admits to recent unprotected sex. What is the likely diagnosis and causative organism?

Lymphogranuloma venereum caused by *C. trachomatis* (LI, L2, L3)

CHAPTER 16

Minor Bacterial Pathogens (*Ehrlichia/ Anaplasma, Moraxella, Haemophilus ducreyi*)

EHRLICHIA CHAFFEENSIS/ANAPLASMA PHAGOCYTOPHILUM

What diseases do *Ehrlichia chaffeensis* and *Anaplasma phagocytophilum* cause?	*Ehrlichia chaffeensis:* monocytic ehrlichiosis *Anaplasma phagocytophilum:* granulocytic anaplasmosis
How do infections present?	Most cases are asymptomatic, but more severe cases present like Rocky Mountain spotted fever (RMSF) except that the typical rash does not occur (i.e., high fever, headache, and myalgias).
How do cells infected with *these organisms* appear on microscopic examination?	*Ehrlichia chaffeensis* infects monocytes and macrophages, forms a characteristic morula (a mulberry-like inclusion body) in the cytoplasm; *A. phagocytophilum* infects granulocytes, sometimes also with morula.
How are these transmitted?	*Ehrlichia chaffeensis:* through the tick *Amblyomma americanum* (lone star tick) and is classically associated with the white-tailed deer *Anaplasma phagocytophilum:* through ixodid ticks (same as Lyme disease)

MORAXELLA CATARRHALIS

What diseases does *Moraxella catarrhalis* cause?

Otitis media and sinusitis in children (third most common cause in the United States). Bronchitis and pneumonia in older people with chronic obstructive pulmonary disease (COPD) or underlying conditions

How is *M. catarrhalis* infection treated?

Almost all strains produce β-lactamase, so commonly prescribed antibiotics include amoxicillin-clavulanate, second- and third-generation oral cephalosporins, trimethoprim-sulfamethoxazole, and azithromycin.

HAEMOPHILUS DUCREYI

What sexually transmitted disease (STD) is caused by *Haemophilus ducreyi*?

Chancroid, characterized by a painful genital ulcer and often localized lymphadenitis. (*H. Ducreyi* is painful and makes you "cry.")

What is the treatment of *H. ducreyi*?

Treatment is either erythromycin or trimethoprim-sulfamethoxazole (TMP-SMX).

PROPIONIBACTERIUM ACNES

Which bacterium produces a lipase that contributes to the genesis of acne skin infections? What is the treatment?

Propionibacterium acnes. Tetracyclines

SECTION III

Basic Virology

CHAPTER 17

General Principles (Structure, Replication)

How are viruses different from other cellular organisms?	Viruses are not capable of self-replication. They can neither produce their own proteins nor generate energy necessary to replicate.
What type of nucleic acid do viruses have?	Either DNA or RNA but not both

STRUCTURE

How is the shape of the virus described?	In terms of the symmetry of the capsid
What is a viral capsid?	Protein coat surrounding the genomic material that is formed by repeating subunits of capsomers
What is the function of viral capsids?	Viral capsids promote viral assembly, protect the genetic material, and facilitate viral attachment to cells.
What are the possible forms of symmetries in viral capsids?	Icosahedral and helical
What is nucleocapsid?	Genome-capsid complex, which is the packaged form of the viral genome

What is a virion?

The complete virus particle that includes the nucleocapsid plus an envelope for enveloped viruses or just the nucleocapsid for nonenveloped viruses

What structure protects the virus and also facilitates viral attachment to cells?

Viral lipoprotein envelope

Which viruses do not have a lipoprotein envelope?

DNA viruses: parvovirus, adenovirus, polyomaviruses, and papillomaviruses
RNA viruses: picornavirus, calicivirus, and reovirus

What are some advantages of having a lipoprotein envelope?

It allows the virus to replicate without lysing the cell and facilitates avoidance of the immune system.

What are some disadvantages of having a lipoprotein envelope?

Enveloped viruses are generally more sensitive to acid, heat, and detergents. All fecal-oral viruses are nonenveloped.

Where do viruses obtain their lipoprotein envelope?

Viruses obtain their envelopes typically from the cell membrane except the herpesvirus that obtains its envelope from the nuclear membrane and bunyavirus from the golgi.

What protein facilitates attachment of the capsid to the envelope?

Matrix protein

What protein spikes out of the lipoprotein envelope and facilitates attachment to cell surface receptors?

Glycoproteins

REPLICATION

What happens during the eclipse period regarding detectable virus levels?

Viruses become undetectable in the serum and intracellularly as they attach, penetrate, and uncoat the viral genome.

What is the latent period?

Time period starting from adsorption of the virus and ending with detectable *extracellular* virus. Note that the latent period is always longer than the eclipse period because by definition the eclipse period ends with detectable *intracellular* virus.

What are the general steps in viral replication?	Attachment and uncoating, early mRNA/protein synthesis, genome replication, late mRNA/protein synthesis, assembly and release
Name the important host cell receptor for each virus:	
Human immunodeficiency virus (HIV)	CD4
Epstein-Barr virus (EBV)	CD21
Rabies	Presynaptic acetylcholine (Ach) receptor
Where do DNA viruses replicate their genome?	In cell nucleus except poxviruses that replicate in the cytoplasm (they are too big to fit in the nucleus)
Where do RNA viruses replicate their genome?	In cytoplasm, except for retroviruses and orthomyxoviruses
What is the difference between early mRNA/protein synthesis and late mRNA/protein synthesis?	While they can occur simultaneously, early mRNA/protein synthesis functions to help replicate the genome and late mRNA/protein synthesis forms the structure for assembly and release.
Where do DNA viruses synthesize mRNA?	In cell nucleus with host cell DNA-dependent RNA polymerase, except poxviruses, which synthesize mRNA in the cytoplasm using a viral DNA-dependent RNA polymerase
How do single-stranded, positive-sense RNA viruses synthesize mRNA?	From the genome, directly as mRNA
How do retroviruses synthesize mRNA?	They utilize a viral reverse transcriptase to form DNA and then a host cell DNA-dependent RNA polymerase to make mRNA.
How do double- and single-stranded, negative-sense RNA viruses synthesize RNA?	Viral RNA-dependent RNA polymerase since no corresponding host enzyme exists
Which DNA virus uses a reverse transcriptase to replicate its genome?	Hepatitis B virus, a DNA virus, makes an intermediate RNA genome that then uses reverse transcriptase to convert into DNA.

Why are certain viral genome types infectious while others are not?

Viral genomes such as single-stranded, positive-sense RNA viruses and DNA viruses (except poxviruses, which replicate in the cytoplasm, and hepatitis B virus, which has a partially single-stranded genome) are infectious because their genome can synthesize all required viral proteins directly with host enzymes.

What is the importance of viral proteases?

Certain viruses make only one mRNA that gets translated into a single polypeptide. Viral proteases cleave the single polypeptide into multiple polypeptides, allowing multiple proteins to be encoded by a single gene. Proteases are important targets in antiviral therapy.

What is the role of the matrix protein in budding of enveloped viruses?

Matrix protein facilitates interaction of the nucleocapsid with the specific site on the membrane.

Are there persistent productive infections in nonenveloped viruses?

No, nonenveloped viruses must either become latent or cause cell lysis. Only enveloped viruses cause persistent, productive infections via budding.

CHAPTER 18

Classification and Characteristics of Medically Important Viruses

DNA VIRUSES

What are the families of DNA viruses?	Hepadnavirus, herpesvirus, adenovirus, parvovirus, polyomavirus, papillomavirus, and poxvirus. Note that polyomavirus and papillomavirus were former genera in the papovavirus family (which no longer exists) and are now considered separate families.
Which DNA viruses have helical capsid symmetry?	None, all DNA viruses have icosahedral symmetry with the exception of the poxvirus, which has a complex capsid that's neither helical nor icosahedral.
Which DNA viruses are enveloped and where in the cell do they acquire their envelope?	Hepadnavirus (cell membrane), poxvirus (cell membrane), herpesviruses (**nu**clear membrane) **Mnemonic:** Herpesviruses cause **nu**merous vesicles.
Which DNA viruses are nonenveloped?	Parvovirus, adenovirus, polyomavirus, and papillomavirus
Are DNA viruses generally single or double stranded?	Most DNA viruses are double stranded.

Which DNA virus is single stranded?

Parvovirus

Mnemonic: Parvovirus is **par**anormal.

Which DNA viruses have circular DNA?

Polyomaviruses (circular), papilloma-viruses (circular), and hepadnaviruses (partially circular)

What viruses belong in the parvovirus family?

B19 (associated with aplastic anemia and erythema infectiosum *fifth disease* "*slapped cheek*," hydrops fetalis, and is the only single-stranded DNA virus)

What viruses belong in the polyomavirus family?

SV40 (natural host is the rhesus monkey but may be associated with tumor formation in humans), BK virus (associated with various kidney diseases), JC virus (causes progressive multifocal leukoencephalopathy)

What viruses belong in the papillomavirus family?

Human papillomavirus (HPV) strains 16 and 18 are associated with cervical cancer.

What viruses belong in the adenovirus family?

Adenovirus (associated with childhood conjunctivitis as well as respiratory and intestinal infections)

What viruses belong in the hepadnavirus family?

Hepatitis B virus (HBV) (only DNA virus with reverse transcriptase and partially circular genome)

What viruses belong in the herpesvirus family?

Herpes simplex virus type 1 (HSV-1) (usually causes oral herpes *cold sores*), herpes simplex virus type 2 (HSV-2) (usually causes genital herpes and neonatal herpes), varicella-zoster virus (VZV) (causes chickenpox and shingles), cytomegalovirus (CMV) (causes severe congenital infections and infections in immunocompromised patients), Epstein-Barr virus (EBV) (causes infectious mononucleosis and associated with nasopharyngeal carcinoma, Burkitt lymphoma, and primary central nervous system [CNS] lymphomas), human herpesvirus 6 (HHV6) (causes roseola infantum *sixth disease*), human herpesvirus 8 (HHV8) (associated with Kaposi sarcoma)

What viruses belong in the poxvirus family?	Smallpox (genome replicates in cytoplasm), vaccinia (causes cowpox and historic source of smallpox vaccine), molluscum contagiosum, and monkeypox
What viral-encoded enzyme enables poxviruses to replicate in the cytoplasm?	Viral DNA-dependent RNA polymerase. Host DNA-dependent RNA polymerase is normally found within the cell nucleus only.

RNA VIRUSES

Which RNA viruses have icosahedral capsid symmetry?	The nonenveloped RNA viruses (picornavirus, calicivirus, and reovirus) along with flavivirus, togavirus, and retrovirus **Mnemonic: PCR** while wearing **F**lavorful **R**etro **T**ogas (**P**icornavirus, **C**alcivirus, and **R**eovirus, **F**lavivirus, **R**etrovirus, **T**ogavirus)
What does it mean to be a positive-sense RNA virus?	The genomic RNA is just like mRNA and can be directly translated by ribosomes into protein.
What does it mean to be a negative-sense RNA virus?	The genomic RNA cannot be translated directly into protein. Instead, it is first transcribed into a positive-stranded RNA which then is translated into protein.
How does a negative-sense RNA become a positive-sense RNA?	RNA viruses carry an enzyme in their capsid called RNA-dependent RNA polymerase, which will transcribe negative-stranded RNA into positive-stranded RNA.
Which positive-sense RNA viruses have linear RNA genomes?	**Retro**viruses, **toga**viruses, **cali**civiruses, **pic**ornoviruses, **flav**iviruses, and coronaviruses. All positive-stranded RNA viruses have linear RNA genomes. **Mnemonic: PC** **F**lavorful **R**etro **T**ogas make **positive** sense.
Which negative-sense RNA viruses have circular RNA genomes? Which ones have linear RNA genomes?	**B**unyaviruses, **a**renaviruses, **d**eltaviruses are circular. **P**aramyxovirus, **r**habdoviruses, **o**rthomyxoviruses, **f**iloviruses are linear. **Mnemonic:** A **BAD PROF** makes **negative** sense.

Which RNA virus has a double-stranded RNA genome?

Reovirus. All other RNA viruses have single-stranded RNA genomes.

Mnemonic: DOUBLE down at the **Reo** Casino

Which viruses are segmented?

Reoviruses, orthomyxoviruses, bunyaviruses, arenaviruses. There are no segmented DNA viruses.

Mnemonic: The island of **BORA BORA** is **segmented.**

Which RNA viruses are enveloped?

Arenaviruses, bunyaviruses, coronaviruses, deltaviruses, filoviruses, flaviviruses, orthomyxoviruses, paramyxoviruses, retroviruses, rhabdoviruses, togaviruses

Which RNA viruses are nonenveloped?

Picornaviruses, caliciviruses, reoviruses

Mnemonic: Naked viruses are easier to **PCR.**

What viruses belong in the picornavirus family?

Polio (causes poliomyelitis), echo (causes meningitis, encephalitis, and common colds), rhino (common cause of cold), coxsackie (causes hand-foot-mouth disease and pericarditis), hepatitis A virus (HAV) (causes oral-fecal hepatitis)

Mnemonic: PERCH

What viruses belong in the calicivirus family?

Norwalk virus (common cause of adult diarrhea)

Mnemonic: Norwalk is a city in **California.**

What viruses belong in the reovirus family?

Reovirus (respiratory enteric orphan virus), rotavirus (leading cause of fatal infantile gastroenteritis)

What viruses belong in the flavivirus family?

Yellow fever (associated with councilman bodies), West Nile, dengue, St Louis encephalitis, Japanese encephalitis, hepatitis C virus (HCV) (hepatitis associated with cirrhosis)

Mnemonic: Did You C Places? (Dengue, Yellow fever, HCV, **Places: West Nile, St Louis, Japan**)

What viruses belong in the togavirus family?

Rubella and the alpha viruses (western/ eastern equine encephalitis)

What viruses belong in the retrovirus family?

Human immunodeficiency virus type 1 (HIV-1) and human immunodeficiency virus type 2 (HIV-2) (genome replicates in nucleus), human T-lymphotrophic virus type 1 (HTLV-1) (associated with adult leukemia) and human T-lymphotrophic virus type 2 (HTLV-2)

What viruses belong in the orthomyxovirus family?

Influenza (genome replicates in nucleus and lacks 5′-capping activity)

What viruses belong in the paramyxovirus family?

Measles virus (has one serotype), mumps virus (has one serotype), respiratory syncytial virus (RSV) (respiratory infections in adults and children), parainfluenza (causes croup)

What viruses belong in the rhabdovirus family?

Rabies virus (associated with Negri bodies and bullet-shaped inclusions in cytoplasm)

What viruses belong in the filovirus family?

Ebola virus, Marburg virus

What viruses belong in the coronavirus family?

Coronavirus (common cause of cold in winter/spring and of severe acute respiratory syndrome [SARS])

What viruses belong in the arenavirus family?

Lymphocytic choriomeningitis virus (has ambisense RNA)

What viruses belong in the bunyavirus family?

California encephalitis, Hantavirus

What viruses belong in the deltavirus family?

Hepatitis delta virus

CHAPTER 19

Pathogenesis and Host Defense (Interferons, Nonspecific and Specific Immunity)

PATHOGENESIS

How do viruses cause cell death?	By taking over the cellular machinery (e.g., ribosomes) so the cells cannot continue to perform necessary functions (e.g., maintenance of membranes, structural proteins, and so on), or by building up virus particles within the cell to cause lysis
How can virus-infected cells be detected by microscope?	Detection of characteristic features such as inclusion bodies (dark concentration of viral particles within the nucleus or cytoplasm), multinucleated giant cells (fused cells), or detection of the cytopathic effect (rounding and darkening of cell). However, many infected cells look identical to normal uninfected cells under the microscope. Direct fluorescent antibodies against viral antigens may help distinguish infected cells.

How do viruses cause signs and symptoms in patients?	By directly killing the cells in which they infect, viruses can cause a whole range of clinical symptoms, depending on the role of the cell. However, for certain viruses, the body's immune response causes disease by killing infected cells (e.g., hepatitis B virus itself causes no cytopathic effect, but cytotoxic T cells kill infected hepatocytes) or activating cytokines that cause generalized symptoms (e.g., influenza).
What are some of the main ways viruses infect the body?	Via the respiratory tract, gastrointestinal (GI) tract, sexually, direct implantation (via trauma), infusions (intravenous [IV] drug abuse or blood transfusions), or transplacental
What is the difference between vertical and horizontal transmissions?	Vertical transmission occurs between mother and newborn; horizontal transmission occurs between two individuals.

NONSPECIFIC IMMUNITY

What are the most important nonspecific first-line defenses?	Interferons and natural killer (NK) cells
How do interferons work?	They inhibit various stages of viral replication by inducing specific anti-viral proteins that cleave viral mRNA, suppress protein synthesis, and increase expression of major histocompatibility complex class I (MHC I) molecules.
Do interferons act intracellularly?	No. They bind to receptors on the cell membrane to initiate production of the antiviral proteins.
What are some important implications of this mechanism?	First, interferons generate a nonspecific antiviral response that is only active in virally infected cells. Second, the antiviral proteins specifically cleave viral mRNA but not host mRNA. Third, interferons cannot act on viruses in the extracellular environment.

What are the types of interferons?	α- and β-Interferons are important in antiviral responses, stimulation of NK cells and macrophages, and play a role in tumor suppression. γ-Interferon has weaker antiviral and antitumor effects but serves to enhance the response to α- and β-interferons by increasing MHC I and II expressions and antigen presentation in all cells.
What are some examples of interferon treatment?	Interferons can be used to treat chronic viral infections such as hepatitis C or chronic hepatitis B. Certain cancers are also susceptible to interferon treatment (e.g., Kaposi sarcoma and hairy cell leukemia).
What type of cell are NK cells? How do NK cells work? Which glycoprotein is most often associated with NK cells?	Lymphocyte NK cells cause apoptosis in cells without MHC I molecules. Viral-infected cells or tumor cells often suppress MHC I molecules in an attempt to evade the immune system. CD56 is the glycoprotein most often associated with NK cells.

SPECIFIC IMMUNITY

What are two important specific immune defenses against viruses?	1. Antibodies 2. CD8 cytotoxic T lymphocytes
What are the two main mechanisms that antibodies utilize to inhibit viruses?	1. Binds to virus receptors on cell surfaces to block viral entry 2. May also lead to lysis of virally infected cells
How else can virally infected cells be lysed?	CD8 T lymphocytes can recognize viral antigen bound to MHC I molecules and activate the FAS protein, leading to apoptosis or release of perforins and granzymes that directly destroy the cell.

What is the difference between active and passive immunities?

Active immunity is the development of antibodies by the immune system in response to viral antigens (either from an infection or vaccine). Passive immunity is the administration of serum containing preformed antibodies against a specific virus or transfer of antibodies from mother to infant. Active immunity provides long-term protection while passive immunity provides only temporary protection.

CHAPTER 20

Viral Drugs and Vaccines

INHIBITORS OF VIRAL ENTRY

What is the mechanism by which amantadine and rimantadine inhibit cell entry of influenza A?

Amantadine and rimantadine inhibit the ion channel function of the influenza A M2 protein. This prevents the pH-dependent step of viral uncoating during endocytosis.

Why is rimantadine used more widely than amantadine?

Amantadine has central nervous system (CNS) side effects. Rimantadine, as a derivative of amantadine, acts via the same mechanism but with fewer side effects. However, both drugs are infrequently indicated due to the high rates of resistance.

What is the mechanism of action of enfuvirtide that blocks fusion of human immunodeficiency virus (HIV)?

Blocks entry of HIV by inhibiting glycoprotein 41 (gp41)-mediated fusion with the CD4 cell membrane

INHIBITORS OF DNA POLYMERASE

What nucleoside inhibitor is widely used to treat herpesvirus infections?

Acyclovir is used to treat herpes simplex virus type 1 (HSV-1), herpes simplex virus type 2 (HSV-2), varicella-zoster virus (VZV), and Epstein-Barr virus (EBV). However, it has no effect on latent HSV and VZV.

127

What is the mechanism of action of acyclovir?

Acyclovir is a guanosine nucleoside analog that is phosphorylated by viral thymidine kinase. After phosphorylation, it competes with deoxyguanosine triphosphate (dGTP) for binding to the viral DNA polymerase and thus prevents further elongation of the DNA.

How does acyclovir achieve its selectivity?

Acyclovir is highly selective because it must be phosphorylated by a virally encoded thymidine kinase to become activated. Activated acyclovir also preferentially inhibits viral DNA polymerase.

What is selective toxicity?

The extent to which a drug can inhibit viral replication without damaging the host cell

Does acyclovir affect recurrences of the herpesvirus after treatment?

No. While it reduces recurrences during treatment, it does not affect latency once treatment is stopped.

How does acyclovir differ from ganciclovir in terms of its clinical use?

Ganciclovir is similar to acyclovir as it is also a guanosine nucleoside analog, but it is more active against cytomegalovirus (CMV). It is activated by a phosphokinase encoded by CMV. It is used to treat the retinitis caused by CMV in AIDS patients as well as other CMV infections.

What is the main non-nucleoside inhibitor of herpesvirus?

Foscarnet

What is the mechanism of action of foscarnet against herpesvirus?

It is a pyrophosphate analog. It binds at the pyrophosphate cleavage site of DNA polymerase and prevents removal of phosphate from the nucleoside triphosphate. This ultimately inhibits the extension of the DNA strand. Foscarnet also inhibits viral RNA polymerase.

Does foscarnet have to be activated by tyrosine kinase or other kinases?

No. Foscarnet is active in vitro and does not require activation by a kinase. It is used in acyclovir-resistant strains of HSV or ganciclovir-resistant strains of CMV. However, not all resistant HSV or CMV will be sensitive to foscarnet because resistance may have developed from mutations in the kinase or DNA polymerase. Mutations in DNA polymerase may also confer resistance to foscarnet.

INHIBITORS OF REVERSE TRANSCRIPTASE

What is highly active antiretroviral therapy (HAART)?

Regimen of three to four anti-HIV drugs that usually consists of two nucleoside reverse transcriptase inhibitors (NRTIs) plus one or two protease inhibitors (PIs) or a non-nucleoside reverse transcriptase inhibitor (NNRTI)

How effective is HAART?

Very effective in reducing mortality and morbidity in compliant patients. However, patients have a quick return to viremia if they stop treatment.

What is the prototype for nucleoside inhibitor of reverse transcriptase?

Zidovudine, also known as azidothymidine (AZT)

What is the mechanism of action of AZT?

It inhibits viral RNA-dependent DNA polymerase (reverse transcriptase) by incorporating into the DNA chain to form a phosphodiester bond with the incoming nucleotide and causes chain termination because it lacks a functional $3'$ hydroxyl group.

Unlike acyclovir, why does AZT have significant adverse side effects?

While acyclovir is phosphorylated by viral thymidine kinase exclusively, AZT is phosphorylated by normal host-cell kinases, so it is activated in all cells.

List some other NRTIs, their indications, and their side effects:

Didanosine (ddI, Videx): deoxyadenosine analog is usually prescribed in combination with other NRTIs; common side effects include pancreatitis, peripheral neuropathy, hyperuricemia, and rarely mitochondrial toxicity leading to lactic acidosis (associated with all NRTIs).

Zalcitabine (ddC, Hivid): cytosine analog is usually prescribed in combination; common side effects include peripheral neuropathy and oral ulcerations.

Stavudine (d4T, Zerit): thymidine analog that is not generally used with AZT because it may reduce phosphorylation of stavudine; main side effects are peripheral neuropathy and stomatitis.

Lamivudine (3TC, Epivir): cytosine analog that is very effective when used with AZT and can also be used for the treatment of chronic hepatitis B infections; well tolerated with minimal side effects such as headache and dizziness.

Abacavir (ABC, Ziagen): guanosine analog that is significantly more effective than other NRTIs; associated with fatal hypersensitivity reactions in 2% to 5% of patients, but sensitivity can be reasonably predicted with genetic analysis (HLA B 5701).

Tenofovir (Viread): belongs to a newer class of nucleotide reverse transcriptase inhibitor (NtRTI); less side effects because it does not require conversion of nucleoside to nucleotide, but most common side effects include nausea, diarrhea, vomiting, and flatulence.

What is the mode of action of NNRTIs?

They inhibit the reverse transcriptase by binding near its active site and inducing a conformational change. They are noncompetitive inhibitors of reverse transcriptase.

What are some NNRTI drugs available in the United States?

1. Nevirapine, efavirenz (first generation)
2. Rilpivirine, etravirine, and doravirine (second generation)

What are the main considerations to use NNRTI as treatment?

They should be used in combination and never as monotherapy. Resistance occurs rapidly and one mutation leads to cross-resistance to other first-generation NNRTIs.

INHIBITORS OF PROTEASE

What is the mode of action of viral protease inhibitors (PI)? Should they be used as monotherapy?

They bind to the active site of HIV protease via specific peptide bonds. The protease therefore cannot cleave the viral precursor. Protease inhibitors should not be used as monotherapy. They leave the proviral DNA unaffected, which means that they cannot suppress the virus on their own.

What are some PIs available in the United States?

Boosted darunavir and atazanavir most commonly used. Regimens are "boosted" by including small doses of ritonavir or cobicistat, which inhibits the metabolism of the other drugs. Less commonly used include lopinavir, indinavir, nelfinavir, saquinavir, and fosamprenavir.

What are the side effects of PIs?

Nausea, diarrhea, hepatotoxicity, skin reactions. Atazanavir can cause renal stones and kidney injuries.

OTHER ANTIVIRALS

What are two antiviral drugs that are used against influenza A and B to inhibit cell-to-cell transmission? What is their mode of action?

1. Zanamivir (Relenza)
2. Oseltamivir (Tamiflu)

They inhibit neuraminidase on the surface of the virus and decrease the ability of the influenza virus to be released from infected cells.

What new antiviral drug blocks influenza proliferation by inhibiting the initiation of mRNA synthesis?

Baloxavir. Approved in the United States in October 2018 and associated with shorter median duration of virus detection than placebo or oseltamivir.

What is the antiviral drug that is used against respiratory syncytial virus (RSV) and what is its mechanism of action?

Ribavirin. It is a guanosine analog that must be phosphorylated to have antiviral activity. It is thought to interfere with guanosine triphosphate (GTP) synthesis, inhibit capping of viral mRNA, and inhibit viral RNA polymerase. It is active against a wide range of viruses, including influenza A, hepatitis C virus (HCV), RSV, and parainfluenza virus.

What is an important side effect of ribavirin?

Hemolytic anemia in 10% of patients

PROPHYLAXIS

What drugs are used to prevent HIV infection in a neonate?

AZT and nevirapine

What drugs are used after an HIV needlestick injury?

AZT, lamivudine, and indinavir or nelfinavir or tenofovir. The regimen is individualized depending on the source patient's history of antiretroviral exposure and resistance.

What is the risk of HIV infection from a hollow-bore needlestick injury from an infected patient?

1/300

VIRAL VACCINES

What types of viral vaccines induce active immunity?

Live-attenuated and killed (inactivated) virus vaccines

What are subunit vaccines?

Subunit vaccines consist of purified protein viral components. They are similar to killed vaccines in that they do not induce a cytotoxic T-cell response.

Name the live-attenuated viral vaccines:

Sabin polio (oral polio vaccine [OPV]), influenza (intranasal), VZV, measles-mumps-rubella (MMR vaccine), yellow fever, smallpox

Mnemonic: Some **F**eeble **V**iruses **M**ay **Y**et **S**trike (**S**abin polio, **F**lu, **V**ZV, **M**MR, **Y**ellow fever, **S**mallpox)

Name the killed inactivated viral vaccines:

Salk polio (inactivated polio vaccine [IPV]), hepatitis A virus (HAV), influenza (IM), rabies

Mnemonic: Salk **H**as **I**nfluenced **R**x (prescriptions) (**S**alk polio, **H**AV, **I**nfluenza, **R**abies)

Name some subunit vaccines:

Hepatitis B, influenza A, HPV

What are the advantages of live viral vaccines?

1. Since the virus multiplies in the host, it produces a CD8 cytotoxic T-cell response.
2. Vaccines given by the natural route of infection induce an immunoglobulin G (IgG) and immunoglobulin A (IgA) response.
3. Live viral vaccines are contagious and may spread immunity to people who were never vaccinated.
4. Live viral vaccines produce a response that is stronger and longer and often confer lifelong protection.

What are the disadvantages of live viral vaccines?

1. Live viral vaccines *can revert to virulence* and cause the very disease they are meant to prevent.
2. Live viral vaccines that do not revert can still cause disease in immunocompromised patients and are relative contraindications.
3. The virus from live viral vaccines can spread to other people and hence cause disease if the vaccine reverts to virulence or if the patient is immunocompromised.
4. Other viruses can contaminate live viral vaccines (e.g., in the 1960s, live polio vaccine was contaminated with SV40, but no side effects have been detected in humans from SV40 exposure).

What is the only live viral vaccine that has reverted to virulence in the past?

Live polio vaccine (Sabin polio vaccine)

What are the advantages of killed viral vaccines?

1. Contamination less likely since the same process that kills the virus in the vaccine would also kill any contaminants.
2. Do not revert to virulence.
3. Vaccines are heat stable so they can be used in hot climates (important for worldwide vaccine programs targeting the underdeveloped world).

What are the disadvantages of killed viral vaccines?

1. Inactivation process may create a vaccine that generates an inadequate immune response.
2. Since the virus does not multiply, there is no CD8 T-cell response.
3. No IgA response.
4. Shorter duration of immunity, resulting in the need for repeated vaccination or booster.

When are most vaccines given, pre- or postexposure to disease-causing agent?

Preexposure

How is passive immunity conferred?

Administering preformed immune globulins

What is passive-active immunity?

Administering both preformed immune globulins to provide protection in the short term and a viral vaccine to provide protection in the long term

Give two common examples of passive-active immunity:

Patients infected with rabies or hepatitis B virus are given both:

1. Immune globulins
2. Vaccine postexposure

Which vaccines should not be given to patients with a history of anaphylactic reactions to eggs? Why?

Influenza, measles, mumps, and yellow fever vaccines as these are grown in chick embryos

When is varicella-zoster immunoglobulin used?

In patients who may have been exposed to VZV, are not immune, and are immunocompromised or pregnant

What is the concept of herd immunity?

Collective immunity for a group of people. It is attained when a critical percentage of the population has been vaccinated so that unimmunized individuals are also protected.

What two traits must a vaccine absolutely confer to attain herd immunity?

Vaccine must both *prevent transmission* of the disease and *prevent the disease itself.*

SECTION IV

Clinical Virology

CHAPTER 21

Herpesviruses

Name the medically important herpesviruses and one or two important diseases they cause:	Herpes simplex virus type 1 (HSV-1): gingivostomatitis and encephalitis
	Herpes simplex virus type 2 (HSV-2): herpes genitalis and neonatal herpes
	Varicella-zoster virus (VZV): varicella (chickenpox) and zoster (shingles)
	Epstein-Barr virus (EBV): infectious mononucleosis and associated with various cancers (e.g., nasopharyngeal carcinoma and Burkett lymphoma)
	Cytomegalovirus (CMV): cytomegalic inclusion disease, mononucleosis, various diseases in immunocompromised
	Human herpesvirus 6 (HHV6): roseola infantum
	Human herpesvirus 8 (HHV8): associated with Kaposi's sarcoma
	Mnemonic: **H**erpes **V**iruses **C**ause **H**armful **E**ffects (**HSV**, **VZV**, **CMV**, **HHV**, **EBV**).
Describe the morphology of the herpesviruses:	Enveloped, icosahedral nucleocapsids with linear double-stranded DNA genome
Where are the viral proteins and DNA synthesized?	DNA and viral proteins are synthesized in the host nucleus.
What is unique about the herpesvirus envelope?	Envelope is derived from the host nuclear membrane. Most other enveloped viruses obtain their membrane from the cell membrane.

Which herpesviruses infect primarily epithelial cells, have relatively short reproductive cycle, and cause latent infections in neurons?

Alpha herpesviruses, which include HSV-1, HSV-2, and VZV

Which herpesviruses have a relatively long reproductive cycle, often causing infected cells to become enlarged and become latent in a variety of tissue?

Beta herpesviruses, which include CMV and HHV6

Which herpesviruses infect and become latent in primarily lymphoid tissue?

Gamma herpesviruses, which include EBV and HHV8

ALPHA HERPESVIRUSES

Name all of the diseases that HSV-1 can cause:

Gingivostomatitis (vesicular lesions, fever, tender regional lymphadenopathy), pharyngotonsillitis (fever, sore throat, ulcerative lesions with grayish exudates on tonsils and pharynx), herpes labialis (prodromal paidn/tingling, vesicles), keratoconjunctivitis (corneal ulcers), encephalitis (fever, hemorrhagic lesion in temporal lobe), and genital herpes (less common than HSV-2)

How is HSV-1 transmitted?

Most people acquire HSV-1 through direct contact or oral secretions during childhood.

Where does HSV-1 usually become latent?

Trigeminal ganglia

How does primary infection with HSV-1 typically present?

Primary infection usually occurs in childhood and is asymptomatic.

How does HSV-1 reactivation usually present?

Vesicular lesions in oral, labial, and ocular mucosae that is preceded by pain, burning, itching, and paresthesia. Lesions are much less severe than primary infection. Viral shedding of HSV-1 occurs up to 96 hours after onset of symptoms.

How is HSV-1 encephalitis diagnosed clinically? What tests are ordered?

Clinically: fever, confusion, headache

Magnetic resonance imaging (MRI): hemorrhagic lesion in the temporal lobe

Cerebrospinal fluid (CSF): increased red blood cells (RBCs) and viral DNA by polymerase chain reaction (PCR)

Electroencephalogram (EEG): diffuse slowing

Mnemonic: In the **ER, TaP CsF** (**E**EG, **R**BCs, **T**emporal lobe, **P**CR CSF, **C**onfusion, **F**ever)

What is the prognosis for untreated and treated HSV-1 encephalitis?

Untreated patients have up to 70% mortality. Treated patients often have neurological sequelae and 20% mortality.

Is HSV-1 encephalitis common?

Yes, it is the most common cause of sporadic, acute necrotizing encephalitis in the United States. Up to 10% to 20% of all cases of encephalitis are caused by HSV-1.

What painful condition is caused by traumatic implantation of herpesvirus into the hands, as commonly seen in dentists?

Herpetic whitlow

Name three diseases that HSV-2 can cause:

1. Meningitis
2. Genital herpes, neonatal herpes
3. Less commonly oral herpes

How is HSV-2 usually transmitted?

Through sexual contact. Lifetime seroprevalence estimates range from 20% to 80%.

Where does HSV-2 usually become latent?

Sacral root ganglia

How does primary infection with HSV-2 typically present?

Primary infections are typically more severe than recurrent outbreaks. Primary episode of genital herpes may last 2 to 3 weeks with painful erythematous, vesicular lesions. Patients may also have asymptomatic primary infections and develop recurrent disease months to years later.

How does HSV-2 reactivation usually present?

Milder outbreak with prodrome of pain, itching, tingling, burning, or paresthesia followed by vesicular lesions. Note that half of HSV-2 seropositive individuals do not have clinically apparent outbreaks but still have episodes of viral shedding and can transmit disease.

Is neonatal herpes a serious infection?

Yes. Cases range from asymptomatic to severe disseminated disease or encephalitis. Ninety percent of neonatal herpes is transmitted perinatally (especially if mother's primary infection was during the pregnancy) and 70% of mothers are asymptomatic. Without therapy, mortality can approach 65%.

How can neonatal herpes be prevented?

Cesarean section, although its routine prophylactic use remains controversial. Only used when there are active symptoms of HSV infection or prodromal symptoms.

What is the Tzanck smear?

A rapid test with Giemsa stain to show multinucleated giant cells. Tzanck smear cannot distinguish between HSV-1, HSV-2, and VZV.

Is it possible to distinguish between HSV-1 and HSV-2?

Yes, with fluorescent antibody or with restriction enzyme cleavage to yield distinct DNA patterns

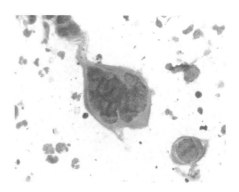

Figure 21.1   Positive Tzanck smear (note large multinucleated keratinocyte). (*With permission from Wolff K, Johnson R.* Fitzpatrick's Color Atlas and Synopsis of Clinical Dermatology. *6th ed. New York, NY: McGraw-Hill; 2009.*)

What is HSV thymidine kinase? How is this important for latency?

Enzyme synthesized by HSV that allows the virus to grow in cells lacking high concentrations of phosphorylated nucleic acid precursors. It converts the nucleotide thymidine to the substance thymidine 5'-phosphate. Neural cells usually do not replicate their genome so they naturally have very low concentrations of these precursors.

How is thymidine kinase pharmacologically important?

Thymidine kinase is necessary to phosphorylate acyclovir into its active form. This is how acyclovir achieves its specificity for HSV.

What diseases does VZV cause? How is chickenpox differentiated from smallpox?

Varicella (chickenpox) and zoster (shingles). Chickenpox has asynchronous vesicles, occurs primarily on the trunk, and the lesions are more superficial. Smallpox has vesicles that are all at the same stage, occurs primarily on the face, arms, and hands, and the mucus membranes of the nose and mouth. Chickenpox is contagious before symptoms appear and smallpox is most contagious after symptoms appear.

What is zoster?

Painful vesicular rash that occurs along a dermatome as a result of reactivation of VZV that lies dormant in the nerve tissue. Zoster can occur in any patient infected with varicella-zoster. The risk of zoster increases with age and impaired immune function.

How might varicella-zoster present in immunocompromised patients?

Immunocompromised patients might develop zoster multiplex (zoster in more than one dermatome), zoster sine herpete (dermatome pain without cutaneous vesicles), myelitis (central nervous system [CNS] deficits), or keratitis (zoster in the ophthalmic division of the trigeminal nerve).

What complication is associated with aspirin administration following influenza B or varicella-zoster virus infection?

Reye syndrome: coma, microvesicular fatty liver, encephalopathy (see Chapter 23)

Where does varicella-zoster usually become latent?	Dorsal root ganglia
What is the treatment of varicella-zoster infections?	Acyclovir or valcyclovir is used for active cases and for prophylaxis in immunocompromised patients.
Is there a vaccine available against chickenpox?	Yes. Both live-attenuated VZV vaccine and VZV immune globulin are available.

BETA HERPESVIRUSES

Name all the diseases that CMV can cause:	Heterophile-negative (aka Monospot negative) mononucleosis syndrome, cytomegalic inclusion disease, and a range of diseases in immunocompromised patients (pneumonia, hepatitis, encephalitis, retinitis, neuropathy, colitis, and CMV syndrome)
How common is CMV infection?	More than 80% of adults have antibodies to CMV.
What is cytomegalic inclusion disease?	Congenital clinical syndrome from CMV infection with multinucleated giant cells, resulting in jaundice, splenomegaly, thrombocytopenia, mental retardation, sensorineural deafness, periventricular calcifications, and microcephaly. Congenital CMV infections do not always develop into inclusion disease.
Is congenital CMV infection common?	Yes. It is the most common cause of congenital abnormalities. Neurological problems such as mental retardation may be present without other signs of CMV infection.
During what trimester of pregnancy is the fetus most at risk for congenital abnormalities from CMV infection?	First trimester, when organs are still developing. The fetus is more at risk if mother has primary infection with CMV during pregnancy.

Why is CMV important in transplant patients?

CMV can cause devastating disease to the immunocompromised transplant patient both directly and by increasing degree of immunodeficiency. CMV pneumonia once had a mortality rate of 85% in marrow transplant patients. It is still one of the most common causes of death in bone marrow transplant patients.

What is the most common manifestation of CMV in human immunodeficiency virus (HIV) patients?

CMV retinitis occurs in 20% to 30% of patients with CD4 count lower than 50 cells/μL.

Pathology Correlate: What is the characteristic finding in cell culture and infected tissue that shows CMV infections?

Owl's-eye nuclear inclusion bodies

Pathology Correlate: What head imaging finding suggests CMV infection?

Periventricular calcifications

How are CMV infections treated?

The drug of choice is ganciclovir (nucleoside analogue that inhibits DNA synthesis). Also available are foscarnet (DNA chain inhibitor of phosphorylation) and cidofovir (nucleoside analogue that inhibits DNA replication)

Name the disease caused by HHV6:

Roseola infantum (sixth disease)

What is roseola infantum?

Clinical syndrome of abrupt onset of high fever for 3 to 5 days followed by an erythematous maculopapular rash sparing the face that appears with the return of normal temperature

Who does HHV6 affect? How is it usually transmitted?

Ninety percent seropositivity is reported in children older than 2 years of age and is transmitted via the saliva of the parents.

What other complications are associated with HHV6?

HHV6 is also the most common cause of febrile seizures in childhood. Also, HHV6 plays a role in HIV patients as it accelerates progression toward AIDS.

GAMMA HERPESVIRUSES

Name the diseases that EBV causes:

EBV causes infectious mononucleosis. It is also linked to lymphoproliferative disorders and tumors such as nasopharyngeal carcinoma and Burkitt lymphoma.

What type of cells does EBV primarily infect?

B cells. EBV also remains latent in B cells.

What is infectious mononucleosis? What patient population is often affected?

Self-limiting syndrome of fever, pharyngitis, generalized lymphadenopathy, and hepatosplenomegaly. More frequently affects adolescents and young adults

Mnemonic: **H**erpesvirus **G**otten **F**rom **P**uckering (**H**epatosplenomegaly, **G**eneralized lymphadenopathy, **F**ever, **P**haryngitis)

What other infectious agents cause infectious mononucleosis-like illness?

CMV, HHV6, acute HIV, toxoplasmosis, viral hepatitis, and syphilis

How is EBV infectious mononucleosis differentiated from other mononucleosis?

EBV infections generate immunoglobulin M (IgM) antibodies that agglutinate sheep and horse RBC (heterophile positive). Other mononucleosis-like illnesses are heterophile negative.

What congenital immunodeficiencies are associated with development of EBV-associated lymphoproliferative disorders?

Wiskott-Aldrich syndrome, **A**taxia-telangiectasia, **C**hédiak-Higashi syndrome, and common variable immunodeficiency (**C**VID)

Mnemonic: **W**orry **A**bout **C**ongenital **C**auses of EBV infections

What disease does EBV cause in immunocompromised patients?

Hairy cell leukoplakia, a nonmalignant lesion of the tongue

Which population has the highest incidence of nasopharyngeal carcinoma?

People from southern China and less common in North American Inuits

How are EBV infections diagnosed?

Classically three criteria:
1. Lymphocytosis (at least 10% atypical lymphocytes)
2. Heterophile test
3. Positive serologic test for EBV

What are atypical lymphocytes?	Infected B cells are *not* the atypical ones; they are actually uninfected activated T cells responding to the EBV infection. They are called atypical lymphocytes due to their abnormal shapes.
Is there treatment of EBV infections?	No antiviral drugs or vaccines are available.
What neoplasm is associated with HHV8?	Kaposi sarcoma
What is Kaposi sarcoma?	Kaposi sarcoma is a vascular neoplasm that manifests in the skin and other organs. It usually begins as a red/purple patch that becomes nodular and plaque-like. It is the most common malignancy in AIDS patients.
Does HHV8 definitively cause Kaposi sarcoma?	No, HHV8 is necessary but not sufficient for the development of Kaposi sarcoma. HHV8 inactivates the tumor suppressor gene retinoblastoma protein (RB).
What is the prognosis for Kaposi sarcoma?	Patients usually do not die of Kaposi sarcoma; however, it is usually present at death. Most patients die from associated opportunistic infections.
How is Kaposi sarcoma diagnosed?	Biopsy, HHV8 DNA/RNA detection

CLINICAL VIGNETTES

A 60-year-old male patient who recently received a heart transplant is now complaining of cough, shortness of breath, and fever. Imaging studies show interstitial pneumonia. On a heart muscle biopsy, what is the characteristic lesion?

Basophilic intranuclear inclusions caused by reactivation of cytomegalovirus (CMV), with smaller eosinophilic cytoplasmic inclusion bodies

A young sexually active man presents to you with a 1-year history of vesicular lesions in his genital area, which spontaneously occur and regress. In what ganglia is the virus thought to cause recurrences by remaining latent?

Herpes simplex virus type 2 remains latent in the sacral ganglia and commonly causes genital infections, whereas herpes simplex virus type 1 remains latent in the trigeminal root ganglion and causes recurrent orolabial cold sores.

A 25-year-old man with a history of AIDS presents with red purple plaques on his foot and the tip of his nose. The lesions are caused by a viral infection. Describe the morphology and genome causal organism:

The description above is that of Kaposi sarcoma, which is caused by human herpesvirus 8, an enveloped, icosahedral capsid with double-stranded linear DNA genome.

A female college student presents with fever, sore throat, lethargy, lymphadenopathy, and splenomegaly. What is the likely diagnosis and causative organism?

Infectious mononucleosis caused by Epstein-Barr virus (EBV)

CHAPTER 22

Hepatitis Viruses

What are the five main clinically relevant hepatitis viruses?

1. Hepatitis A
2. Hepatitis B
3. Hepatitis C
4. Hepatitis D
5. Hepatitis E

Mnemonic: HAV causes **P**uking (**P**icornavirus), HBV causes **H**epatitis (**H**epadnavirus), HCV most **F**atal (**F**laviviridae), HDV is **D**eficient (**D**elta virus), HEV is bad for **E**xpectant mothers (**HE**padenavirus)

HEPATITIS A

To what virus family does hepatitis A virus (HAV) belong? Describe its morphology:

Picornavirus. Smallest (27-nm diameter), nonenveloped, icosahedral, single-stranded, positive-sense RNA virus

How many immunological strains of HAV are there? How is HAV transmitted?

Although HAV genome may vary by 20%, there is only one serotype. Infection confers immunity from all HAV strains. HAV is transmitted by fecal-oral route.

How common is HAV infection?

HAV is almost universal in developing nations and in about one-third of adults in the United States have evidence of past infection.

Is there a chronic HAV carrier state?

No. HAV usually causes a self-limited acute reaction with complete recovery.

How is it possible to distinguish between active and past HAV infections?

Active HAV infection is characterized by anti-HAV immunoglobulin M (IgM) and elevated serum aminotransferases. Past HAV infection is characterized by anti-HAV immunoglobulin G (IgG).

How can HAV infection be prevented?

Active immunization with an attenuated vaccine or passive immunization with anti-HAV IgG

In which season do most HAV infections occur?

Autumn

How is HAV transmitted?

Fecal-oral route. Oysters are commonly used as a food of choice on exams.

HEPATITIS B

Hepatitis B virus (HBV) belongs to which family of viruses?

Hepadnavirus

What is unique about the genome of HBV compared to all other hepatitis viruses?

HBV has a partially single-stranded and partially double-stranded DNA genome whereas all other hepatitis viruses have an RNA genome.

What is unique about the replicative strategy of HBV?

HBV relies on an RNA-dependent DNA polymerase (reverse transcriptase [RT]) to replicate its genome.

Describe the replication cycle of HBV:

1. HBV binds to the hepatocyte membrane.
2. Virion uncoats and the DNA genome enters the nucleus.
3. DNA genome gets repaired to form a covalently closed circular DNA (cccDNA).
4. DNA-dependent RNA polymerase forms messenger RNA (mRNA) and pregenomic RNA from cccDNA.
5. Pregenomic RNA, nucleocapsid, polymerase proteins are encapsulated in the virus core particle in cytoplasm.
6. RT forms genomic DNA (double- and single-stranded) within virus core particle.
7. Virus core particle can reinfect the same nucleus to form more cccDNA or be secreted as virion.

How does the function of RT differ between HBV and retroviruses?

RT forms genomic DNA within the viral core particle in HBV. Human immunodeficiency virus (HIV) requires RT to form DNA immediately after fusion. HBV requires RT to form progeny; HIV requires RT to integrate into genome and produce viral proteins.

What is unique about the size of the HBV genome?

HBV has a small (3.2 kb) genome that has four overlapping genes: S encodes hepatitis B surface antigen (HBsAg); C encodes hepatitis B envelope antigen (HBeAg) and hepatitis B core antigen (HBcAg); P codes for DNA polymerase; and X encodes hepatitis B X antigen (HBxAg).

How common is HBV infection? How is HBV transmitted?

More than 350 million are HBV carriers worldwide and approximately 1.2 million HBV carriers in the United States. Vertical (maternal-infant) transmission in endemic areas (Southeast Asia, China, and sub-Saharan Africa). Horizontal (transfusions, sexually, intravenous [IV] drug) transmission in areas of low prevalence

Does HBV cause acute or chronic hepatitis?

Both. Ninety percent of perinatally acquired HBV develop chronic HBV infection whereas less than 5% of immunocompetent adults develop chronic HBV after infection.

How can HBV infection be diagnosed?

Most commonly serologically using HBsAg, but diagnosis can also be obtained using immunohistochemistry, in situ hybridization, or PCR

What are the commonly used serological markers for HBV?

HBsAg, HBeAg, anti-HBc IgM, anti-HBc IgG, anti-HBs (HBsAb), anti-HBe (HBeAb), and HBV DNA

What is the significance of HBsAg?

Presence of HBsAg in serum is diagnostic for HBV infection. HBsAg typically appears in the blood in 1 to 10 weeks after infection. Persistence of HBsAg for over 6 months is diagnostic for chronic HBV infection.

What is the significance of hepatitis B surface antibody (HBsAb)?

HBsAb is protective against HBV infection and detectable HBsAb correlates to resolution of an acute HBV infection, past HBV infection, or successful immunization.

What is the significance of anti-HBc?

Anti-HBc IgM develops before HBsAb and is usually diagnostic for acute HBV infection. Anti-HBc IgM is detectable during the window period. Anti-HBc IgG is indicative of past acute or chronic HBV infection and may persist longer than HBsAb.

What is the window period?

In acute HBV infection, there may be a window period following the disappearance of HBsAg in the serum but before the appearance of HBsAb. During this period, anti-HBc IgM is usually detectable. However, as the laboratory sensitivities for detection of HBsAg and HBsAb have improved, this window period is now rarely clinically significant.

What is the significance of HBeAg?

HBeAg is a marker of HBV replication and infectivity. Anti-HBe may be detected in both patients with acute or chronic HBV infection.

What are clinical serological markers for hepatitis?

Aspartate aminotransferase (AST) and alanine aminotransferase (ALT). In general, viral hepatitis ALT is greater than AST, whereas alcoholic hepatitis AST is greater than ALT.

What is fulminant hepatitis?

Unusual (0.1%–0.5%) outcome following HBV infection that results from massive immune-mediated lysis of infected hepatocytes. More than 50% of all fulminant hepatitis cases are related to HBV but usually with underlying hepatitis D virus (HDV) or hepatitis C virus (HCV) coinfection.

What cancer is associated with HBV infection?

Hepatocellular carcinoma

What is the treatment of HBV infection?

Adult-acquired acute HBV infection usually does not require treatment. Neonates born to HBsAg-positive mothers should receive HBV vaccine and HBsAb immediately following birth. Chronic HBV patients may be treated with α-interferon or lamivudine (RT inhibitor).

Does congenital HBV infection results in acute or chronic infections?

Chronic infections. Infants are less likely to develop acute infections due to not having a fully developed immune system.

Who should get the HBV vaccine?

Everybody should be vaccinated as it has been shown to be safe and cost-effective.

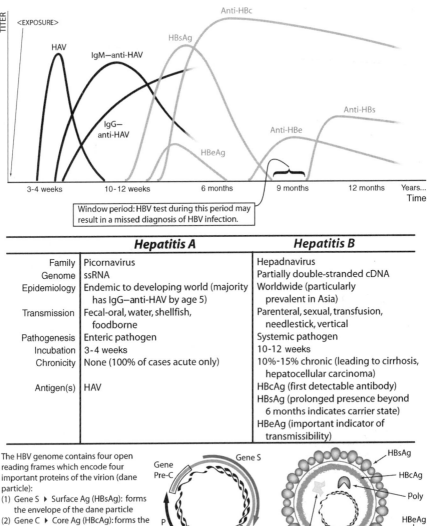

Window period: HBV test during this period may result in a missed diagnosis of HBV infection.

	Hepatitis A	Hepatitis B
Family	Picornavirus	Hepadnavirus
Genome	ssRNA	Partially double-stranded cDNA
Epidemiology	Endemic to developing world (majority has IgG–anti-HAV by age 5)	Worldwide (particularly prevalent in Asia)
Transmission	Fecal-oral, water, shellfish, foodborne	Parenteral, sexual, transfusion, needlestick, vertical
Pathogenesis	Enteric pathogen	Systemic pathogen
Incubation	3-4 weeks	10-12 weeks
Chronicity	None (100% of cases acute only)	10%-15% chronic (leading to cirrhosis, hepatocellular carcinoma)
Antigen(s)	HAV	HBcAg (first detectable antibody) HBsAg (prolonged presence beyond 6 months indicates carrier state) HBeAg (important indicator of transmissibility)

The HBV genome contains four open reading frames which encode four important proteins of the virion (dane particle):
(1) Gene S ▶ Surface Ag (HBsAg): forms the envelope of the dane particle
(2) Gene C ▶ Core Ag (HBcAg): forms the nucleocapsid protein
(3) Gene X ▶ X Protein: the transcription factor
(4) P ▶ DNA Polymerase (poly): has both transcriptase and reverse-transcriptase activities

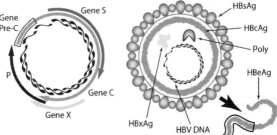

Figure 22.1   Hepatitis A versus hepatitis B.

HEPATITIS C

To what virus family does hepatitis C virus (HCV) belong? Describe its morphology.

Flaviviridae. Spherical (40–60 nm), enveloped, single-stranded, positive-sense RNA virus

How many different genotypes of HCV are there?

At least six genotypes identified. With a rapid mutation rate, there appears to be no effective long-term neutralizing antibodies. Past infection does not confer immunity.

How common is HCV infection?

An estimated 4 million (1.8% of population) in the United States and 170 million worldwide (up to 22% in Egypt). Most have chronic infections. New acute HCV infections are uncommon.

How is HCV usually transmitted?

HCV was associated with 90% of transfusion-related hepatitis prior to 1992 in the United States and was referred to as *non-A, non-B* hepatitis. Since identification, transfusion-related HCV has dramatically decreased and IV drugs use is the most common form of transmission. Sexual and perinatal transmission is also possible but significantly less likely.

What are the chances of acquiring HCV through an accidental needlestick from an HCV-infected patient?

3%

What percentage of acute HCV infections develops into chronic HCV infections?

60% to 80%

How is HCV diagnosed?

Detection of antibodies to HCV polypeptides by anti-HCV-ELISA(90%–95% sensitive) or direct detection of HCV RNA (gold standard)

What are common sequelae of HCV infection?

Cirrhosis (20% after 20 years of HCV infection) and hepatocellular carcinoma (1%–4% per year in HCV cirrhotic patients)

What are the treatments for both acute and chronic HCV infection?	Traditionally were α-interferon and ribavirin. Newer antiviral therapies such as simepravir, sofosbuvir, ledipasvir are associated with long-term sustained virologic response (or cure). Regiment depends on specific genotype.
How can HCV infection be prevented?	Avoid needlesticks, IV drugs, and screen transfusion blood. There is no vaccine available for HCV.

HEPATITIS D

To what virus family does hepatitis D virus (HDV) belong? Describe its morphology:	Delta virus. Defective, single-stranded, negative polarity, circular RNA (smallest genome 1.7 kb)
HDV infection can only occur in the presence of which other virus? Why?	HBV. HDV requires the outer envelope HBsAg for assembly. **Mnemonic:** HDV is **D**efective and therefore needs HBV to help it.
How common is HDV infection?	HDV is endemic among HBV-infected people in the Mediterranean, North Africa, and South America and patients who receive frequent transfusions. Globally 5% of HBV-infected people are coinfected with HDV.
What are important sequelae of HDV infection?	HDV increases the severity of HBV infection and can transform asymptomatic chronic HBV infection into severe chronic hepatitis. HDV is also associated with fulminant hepatitis. However, HDV does not increase the frequency with which acute HBV infection progresses to chronic HBV infection.
Which type of HDV infection is clinically more severe?	HDV superinfection on HBV is more severe than HDV coinfection.
How can you prevent HDV infection?	By HBV vaccine

HEPATITIS E

To what virus family does hepatitis E virus (HEV) belong? Describe its morphology:

Most similar to calcivirus family, although recently, HEV has been classified as its own hepevirus family. Nonenveloped, single-stranded, positive-sense RNA

How is HEV predominately transmitted? Where do HEV infections occur?

Through fecal-oral route. Southeast and Central Asia, the Middle East, and North and West Africa. In the United States, linked to travel to endemic areas

Why is HEV infection particularly bad for pregnant women?

HEV infections in pregnant women have a fatality rate of 15% to 25%, compared to only 1% to 3% overall fatality rate

CLINICAL VIGNETTE

A 32-year-old, 8-month pregnant woman with a history of intravenous drug tells you that she is worried that she has acquired the hepatitis B virus because she shared needles with her partner 10 months ago who is a known carrier of the virus. What marker will you find in the patient's blood if she is a chronic carrier? What marker will you look for to suggest patient is infectious?

Hepatitis B surface antigen (for >6 months), anti-HBc antibodies. There will be no anti-hepatitis B surface antigen antibodies. Hepatitis B envelope antigen presence is suggestive of infectious state.

CHAPTER 23

Paramyxovirus and Orthomyxovirus

What are the similarities between paramyxoviruses and orthomyxoviruses?	Both are enveloped, helical, and negative-sense RNA viruses. Both also tend to spread via the respiratory tract.
What is an important difference between the genome of paramyxoviruses and orthomyxoviruses?	Orthomyxoviruses have a segmented RNA genome that allows for antigenic shifts. Paramyxoviruses have nonsegmented RNA genomes and most only have one serotype, allowing for long-term immunity.
Name some orthomyxoviruses and the common disease they cause:	Influenza A and B viruses. Cause common flu
Name the paramyxoviruses and the common diseases they cause:	Parainfluenza virus (croup, bronchitis, and bronchopneumonia), respiratory syncytial virus (RSV) (pneumonia and bronchiolitis in young infants), measles virus (measles), mumps virus (mumps)

ORTHOMYXOVIRUS

What is unique about the envelope of orthomyxoviruses?	It is covered with two separate long glycoprotein spikes, hemagglutinin (HA) and neuraminidase (NA).
What is the role of hemagglutinin in orthomyxoviruses?	HA attaches to host sialic acid on the surface of upper respiratory tract, allowing for attachment of the virus. It is recognized as one of the major virulence factors associated with influenza. HA causes hemagglutination by agglutinating erythrocytes via sialic acid.

What step of orthomyxovirus infection would be missing if the virus lacked HA?

Adsorption. The virus would not be able to enter the cell.

What is the role of neuraminidase in orthomyxovirus infection?

NA cleaves neuraminic acid and disrupts the mucin barrier. This exposes the sialic acid and facilitates infection of the host cells. NA also helps release progeny virus after a cell has been infected.

How are HA and NA attached to the viral membrane?

They are anchored to the inside of the viral envelope by membrane proteins (M proteins).

What do the M1 and M2 proteins do?

M1 is a membrane protein that provides structural stability under the envelope. M2 is an ion channel that acidifies viral interior to disrupt the structure of M1 and facilitates uncoating of the virus.

How does the drug amantadine work?

Amantadine specifically blocks the M2 protein, thus preventing uncoating of the virus.

How does the influenza vaccine prevent influenza infections?

Influenza vaccine results in antibodies against hemagglutinin

Describe the internal structure of an orthomyxovirus:

Helical capsid with eight-segmented, single-stranded, negative-sense RNA genome

What is unique about influenza genome replication?

Only other RNA virus, besides retroviruses, that has genome synthesis inside the nucleus

How many types of the influenza virus are there?

Three. Influenza A, B, and C

Does the influenza virus infect other organisms besides humans?

Yes. Influenza A is able to infect mammals and birds in addition to humans. Influenza B and C can only infect humans.

In 1918, 20 million people worldwide died from the influenza virus. What is this an example of?

A pandemic (a worldwide epidemic)

Which strains of influenza are involved with pandemics? Why?

Only influenza A causes pandemics. Remember that influenza A is the only strain that infects animals other than humans. This allows for antigenic shift. Influenza B is known to cause outbreaks, while influenza C typically causes mild infections.

Mnemonic: Large to small (A = pandemic, B = epidemic, C = mild infection)

What is the difference between antigenic shift and antigenic drift?

Antigenic shift involves the creation of entirely new strains of influenza based on the exchange of genomic segments between human strains and animal strains. Antigenic drift involves minor mutations in HA or NA that changes the antigenic nature of these glycoproteins.

Mnemonic: Drifting is a slow process, shifting (e.g., earthquakes) is a drastic process.

Why are new versions of the influenza vaccine introduced every year?

Antigenic drift

Who is most likely to suffer serious complications from influenza?

Elderly and immunocompromised hosts

How can infection with influenza contribute to bacterial pneumonia?

The viral infection lowers the host defenses against many bacteria, most notable *Staphylococcus aureus* and *Streptococcus pneumoniae*.

What are the symptoms of Reye syndrome?

Coma, fatty liver, and encephalopathy

Mnemonic: Reyes syndrome, Children Might Expire (Coma, Microvesicular fatty liver, Encephalopathy)

What is the cause of Reye syndrome?

There is evidence that salicylate use in children with influenza and chicken-pox may cause this serious condition. Salicylates (aspirin) should never be given to children to reduce fevers.

What's another medical complication that can arise from influenza infection?

Guillain-Barré syndrome

What laboratory tests could be used to confirm an influenza infection?	Culture (to isolate the virus), detection of viral proteins, detection of viral RNA (reverse transcriptase use followed by polymerase chain reaction [PCR]), and serological tests
What drugs are available to treat influenza?	Commonly zanamivir (inhaled)/ oseltamivir (Tamiflu, oral) that are NA inhibitors. Baloxavir is a novel oral agent that inhibits influenza mRNA synthesis. Amantadine/rimantadine prevent viral replication by blocking the viral M2 protein but is only active against influenza A and has high rates of resistance.
What medicine can be used against influenza B?	Zanamivir, oseltamivir, and baloxavir can be used against both A and B types. They have been shown to be effective in reducing the duration of symptoms and preventing infection.
What is the best way to prevent influenza infection?	Vaccine. Typically contains two killed strains of influenza A and one strain of influenza B

PARAMYXOVIRUS

How are paramyxoviruses different from orthomyxoviruses?	1. The genome is nonsegmented. 2. HA and NA are part of the same glycoprotein spike (except RSV lacks both HA/NA and measles virus lacks NA). 3. Paramyxoviruses have a fusion protein that causes infected host cells to fuse together and become multinucleated giant cells. **Mnemonic:** My **PAiR** of front teeth needed a **SINGLE STRAND** of braces to **FUSE** the gaps together.
How many serotypes do the paramyxoviruses have?	Mumps and measles viruses have only one serotype. Parainfluenza virus has four serotypes and RSV has two serotypes.
How are paramyxoviruses transmitted?	Via respiratory droplets

How does parainfluenza virus typically present in young children?

As croup which is characterized by stridor and a barking cough that is caused by air moving through narrowed upper airways

Are there any drugs or vaccines available for croup?

No

How does RSV differ structurally from other paramyxoviruses?

It lacks both HA and NA glycoproteins.

For what disease in young children RSV is the number one cause? What time of year do RSV outbreaks tend to occur?

Pneumonia. During winter and spring

Pathology Correlate: What laboratory tests are used to confirm infection with RSV?

Immunofluorescence or cell culture (characteristically shows multinucleated giant cells)

How can RSV infections be prevented?

Palivizumab, a monoclonal antibody specific against the fusion protein; or respiratory syncytial virus immune globulin intravenous (human) (RSV-IGIV), a purified polyclonal immunoglobulin against RSV

Does prior infection with RSV generate immunity for life?

No, but a subsequent infection would be limited to the upper respiratory tract

What are the most common clinical findings in patients with mumps?

Fever, malaise, and swelling of the parotids glands. Mumps virus can also cause orchitis and aseptic meningitis.

Mnemonic: Causes **PAiRs** of h**UMPS** (two parotids, two testes, two hemispheres of the brain). **PAR**amyxovirus **MUMPS**

Can mumps be prevented?

Yes. The measles-mumps-rubella (MMR) vaccine, a live-attenuated vaccine, can prevent mumps.

What are the first signs of measles (rubeola)?

Measles prodrome consists of conjunctivitis, swelling of eyelids, photophobia, high fevers, cough, coryza, and malaise. The prodrome is followed by the appearance of Koplik spots (enanthem) and then a 5-day maculopapular rash (exanthema) that spreads from the face to the trunk and extremities.

Mnemonic: 4 C's Coryza (purulent rhinitis), Conjunctivitis, Cough, Koplik spots

What are Koplik spots?

Bluish-white spots on a red base in the buccal, gingival, or labial mucosae that appear before the onset of a maculopapular rash. It is pathognomonic for measles.

Describe the measles rash:

A red, flat to slightly bumpy (maculopapular) rash that spreads from forehead → face → neck → torso → hits feet by day 3. The rash disappears in the same sequence in which it appears and typically is cleared from the face by the time it appears on the feet.

What late sequelae of measles develop up to 20 years after initial measles infection and present as a progressive degenerative neurological disease?

Subacute sclerosing panencephalitis (SSPE)

What is the cause of SSPE? How can SSPE be prevented?

A defective form of measles virus (lack or altered expression of M-matrix protein). It can be prevented with the MMR vaccine.

CLINICAL VIGNETTES

A 3-year-old child presents with a harsh cough and hoarseness. What are the likely diagnosis and causative organism? Describe the morphology and genome of the causative organism:

Croup caused by parainfluenza virus. Enveloped helical capsid with single-stranded, negative polarity RNA genome

A 13-year-old girl died of a progressive degenerative neurologic disease. Her intellect and personality had been deteriorating. She had seizures and a state of decerebrate rigidity. She died 6 months after onset of symptoms. She had a severe attack of measles as a child. What does she have?

Subacute sclerosing panencephalitis (SSPE)

A 7-year-old Hispanic boy presents with cough, runny nose, conjunctivitis, and red lesions with bluish centers in his buccal mucosa. What illness may be suspected based on this classic presentation?

Measles

CHAPTER 24

Arboviruses (Toga, Flavi, Bunya)

What are arboviruses?	Arboviruses (arthropod-borne viruses) are a diverse group of viruses that spread via arthropods (most commonly mosquitoes).
What classification of families are the most commonly considered arboviruses?	Flavivirus, togavirus, bunyavirus **Mnemonic:** Transmitted From Bugs (Toga, Flavi, Bunya)

FLAVIVIRUS

What are the main pathogenic viruses in the flavivirus family?	Yellow fever virus, dengue virus, West Nile virus, hepatitis C virus (HCV), St Louis encephalitis virus, and Japanese encephalitis virus **Mnemonic: Did You C Places?** (Dengue, Yellow fever, HCV, **Places: West Nile, St Louis, Japan**)
Describe the morphology and genome of flaviviruses:	Enveloped, icosahedral capsid with a nonsegmented, single-stranded, positive-sense RNA genome
Where do flaviviruses replicate their genomes?	In the cytoplasm
What are the main vectors for flaviviruses?	*Aedes* mosquito for yellow fever virus and dengue virus. *Culex* mosquito for West Nile virus, St Louis encephalitis virus, and Japanese encephalitis virus **Mnemonic:** Remember to wear your **Rolex** when you see **places**. *Cu*lex (**West Nile, St. Louis, Japan**)

Hepatitis C virus is classified in the flavivirus family. Is it also considered an arbovirus?

No (there are no arthropod vectors for the virus)

What are the symptoms of yellow fever virus?

Initial symptoms include fever/chills, headaches, myalgia, and nausea. Then symptoms progress to high fever, black vomitus (hematemesis), jaundice, albuminuria, and eventually CNS symptoms such as seizures and comas.

Pathology Correlate: What pathological changes can be seen in the liver with yellow fever infections?

Lobular necrosis with Councilman bodies

What are the two vectors for yellow fever virus?

There are two distinct types of yellow fever with two vectors.
1. In jungle yellow fever, *Haemagogus* mosquitoes transmit the virus from monkeys to humans.
2. In urban yellow fever, *Aedes aegypti* transmits the virus between humans.

What type of vaccine is available for this virus?

A live-attenuated viral vaccine

Are there any treatments for yellow fever virus?

No. Mortality is approximately 50%, so prevent yellow fever with vaccine and mosquito control.

What are the symptoms for dengue virus (*break-bone disease*)?

There are two types of dengue fever.
1. Classic dengue fever is characterized by abrupt initial onset with fever and generalized rash that develops into retro-orbital muscle and joint pain.
2. Dengue hemorrhagic fever is characterized by increased vascular permeability (increased hematocrit, ascites, and pleural effusions), thrombocytopenia (bleeding), and abnormal liver function tests.

What is the prognosis for dengue fever?

Classic dengue fever usually resolves and is rarely fatal. Dengue hemorrhagic fever is associated with 3% mortality if treated and 50% mortality if untreated.

What is dengue shock syndrome?	A clinical syndrome that occurs as an extreme form of dengue hemorrhagic fever in which excessive vascular permeability leads to shock. It is associated with a 12% mortality in aggressively treated patients and typically occurs 3 to 7 days after the initial illness.
Is there a vaccine available for this virus?	No. Unfortunately, dengue virus is also spreading in Asia, Africa, and the Americas.
Are infections with the West Nile virus usually symptomatic?	No. About 80% of patients infected with the West Nile virus remain asymptomatic. However, West Nile virus may cause rapidly fatal encephalitis or meningitis (especially in the elderly).
What is the reservoir for West Nile virus?	Wild birds are the main reservoir and it is transmitted to humans by mosquitoes.
What is the prognosis for West Nile virus infection?	Patients with mild infections usually fully recover. However, encephalitis is associated with 12% mortality.
What is the most important way to prevent West Nile virus infection in humans?	Mosquito control since there are no vaccines or effective treatments

TOGAVIRUS

What are the main pathogenic viruses in the togavirus family?	Rubella virus, western and eastern equine encephalitis virus (WEE and EEE)
Describe the morphology and genome of togaviruses:	Enveloped, icosahedral capsid with a nonsegmented, single-stranded, positive-sense RNA genome
Where do togaviruses replicate their genomes?	In the cytoplasm
What are the main vectors for togaviruses?	WEE and EEE are transmitted via mosquitoes. Rubella is transmitted via airborne droplets or congenitally.

What congenital defects are caused by congenital rubella infection?

Heart (patent ductus arteriosus, interventricular septal defects, and pulmonary stenosis), eyes (cataracts and chorioretinitis), CNS (mental retardation, microcephaly, and deafness), and skin (blueberry muffin rash)

What percentage of newborns born to women infected with rubella during the first trimester of pregnancy develops congenital rubella?

25%. Defects are rare if infection occurs after the 20th week of pregnancy.

What is the best test for rubella in a pregnant woman?

Immunoglobulin M (IgM) antibody titer indicates recent infection. Amniocentesis can test if virus is in the amniotic fluid, which is confirmatory for fetal infection.

What is the best way to prevent congenital rubella?

Live-attenuated vaccine (measles-mumps-rubella [MMR] vaccine). However, unimmunized pregnant women should not receive the MMR vaccine.

What are the clinical findings for noncongenitally acquired rubella?

Mild fever and rash (from forehead to face to torso to extremities)

How is noncongenitally acquired rubella contracted?

Respiratory secretions

What is another name for noncongenital rubella?

German measles or 3-day measles

How do you differentiate between rubella and measles?

Rubella is typically mild and lasts only 3 days. Measles characteristically lasts 5 to 7 days with rashes that begin on the face, spread toward the trunk, and eventually to the extremities. Rubella presents with generalized lymphadenopathy while measles more commonly presents with cervical lymphadenopathy.

What are the clinical findings for the equine encephalitis viruses?

Headache, fever, altered level of consciousness, and focal neurological deficits

What is the reservoir for equine encephalitis viruses?

Wild birds

Besides humans, name another host for the equine encephalitis viruses.

Horses

BUNYAVIRUS

What are the main pathogenic viruses in the bunyavirus family?

Hantavirus, California encephalitis, and Rift Valley fever virus

What type is the morphology and genome of bunyaviruses?

Enveloped helical capsid with segmented (three segments), single-stranded, negative-sense RNA genome

Where do bunyaviruses replicate their genomes?

In the cytoplasm

Mnemonic: Bunya **R**eplicate **H**appily in **C**ytoplasm (**R**ift **V**alley, **H**anta, **C**alifornia).

What are the symptoms of Hantavirus?

Hantavirus can present as Hantavirus cardiopulmonary syndrome (fever, bilateral diffuse interstitial edema, development within 72 hours of hospitalization) and hemorrhagic fever with renal syndrome (fever, hemorrhage, hypotension, renal failure).

What is the reservoir for Hantavirus?

Deer mouse

What is the most common way to acquire Hantavirus in the United States?

Inhalation of dried rodent feces. Patients commonly will have a history of indoor exposure to rodent-infested buildings.

What is the prognosis with Hantavirus cardiopulmonary syndrome infection?

Poor. During the 1993 outbreak in the Four Corners region mortality reached 80%. Mortality rate is now approximately 40%.

What is the prognosis with Hantavirus hemorrhagic fever with renal syndrome?

Less than 5% mortality. Although hemorrhagic fever with renal syndrome is much more common than Hantavirus cardiopulmonary syndrome

What is California encephalitis?

An encephalitis, first identified in California in 1946 that although has a low (<1%) mortality, is known to leave 20% of infected patients with recurrent seizures.

What is Rift Valley fever?

A flu-like illness infecting people and domestic animals in sub-Saharan Africa commonly associated with mosquito epidemics in years with heavy rainfall. Patients may also develop hemorrhagic fever, encephalitis, and ocular damage (1%–10% with permanent vision loss).

What is the vector for California encephalitis and Rift Valley fever?

Mosquitoes

CLINICAL VIGNETTES

A 25-year-old man returned from an *Aedes* mosquito–infested area in Africa a week ago and presents with high fever, jaundice, and black vomitus. What virus most likely caused his symptoms?

Yellow fever virus

A 30-year-old woman returned from an *Aedes* mosquito–infested area in Central America a week and a half ago and presents with fever, chills, headache, myalgia, and deep bone pain in the back. What virus most likely caused her symptoms?

Dengue virus

A 67-year-old woman living in Southern California with stagnant water nearby presents initially with fever, lymphadenopathy, and rash, which soon progresses to meningitis followed by death due to encephalitis. A dead crow was seen on her lawn a week before the onset of illness. What virus most likely caused her death?

West Nile virus

This virus preferentially replicates in the motor neurons of the anterior horn of the spinal cord. While infection is often asymptomatic, flaccid paralysis including life-threatening respiratory paralysis can occur. What is this virus?

Poliovirus (and West Nile virus)

A newborn child presents with a machinery-like murmur heard throughout systole and diastole between the shoulder blades. Which congenitally acquired infection is most likely suspected?

Rubella

A 22-year-old man living in New Mexico presents with influenza-like symptoms and suddenly develops pulmonary edema. The patient requires mechanical ventilation to enhance oxygenation. After 9 days, the patient succumbs to the illness and dies. What virus should be suspected?

Hantavirus (Hantavirus pulmonary syndrome)

CHAPTER 25

Retroviruses

What enzyme do all retroviruses possess and what is the function of the enzyme?	Reverse transcriptase. It is an RNA-dependent DNA polymerase that transcribes viral RNA into DNA.
Which other family of viruses utilizes reverse transcriptase?	Hepadnaviruses (HBV)
Describe the general structure of retroviruses:	Enveloped, icosahedral capsid
Describe the steps of retroviral replication:	1. Binding of virus to receptor on host cell
	2. Fusion of virus to host cell membrane and entry of viral material
	3. Transcription of viral RNA by reverse transcriptase into double-stranded DNA
	4. Integration of viral DNA into host DNA
	5. Transcription of viral DNA by host RNA polymerase into messenger RNA (mRNA)
	6. Translation of viral mRNA by host polymerases
	7. Cleavage of viral proteins by viral and host proteases
	8. Budding from the host cell membrane
What are the two medically important retroviruses?	1. Human immunodeficiency virus (HIV)
	2. Human T-cell lymphotropic virus 1 (HTLV-1)

| How do HIV and HTLV affect host cells differently? | HIV kills T cells, while HTLV does not. Instead, HTLV causes transformations in T cells that allow them to proliferate uncontrollably. |

RETROVIRAL GENETICS

Are retroviruses diploid or haploid?	Diploid. They are the only family of viruses that are diploid.
Describe the genome of retroviruses:	Single-stranded, positive-polarity RNA genome
What are the three genes common to all retroviruses?	*gag*, *pol*, and *env*
What does the *gag* gene encode for?	Internal core and matrix proteins, including protein 24 and protein 17 (p24 and p17)
What does the *pol* gene encode for?	Several enzymes, including reverse transcriptase, protease, and integrase
What does the *env* gene encode for?	p160, which is cleaved to form two surface proteins, glycoprotein 120 and glycoprotein 41 (gp120 and gp41) in HIV or gp46 and gp21 in HTLV
What is the function of protease?	Cleaves polyproteins encoded by the *pol* and *gag* genes
When does protease cleave the *pol* and *gag* polyproteins?	When the virus buds from the host cell membrane
Why is the cleavage of *pol* and *gag* important?	Virus becomes mature and infectious after cleavage.
What is the function of integrase?	Integrates viral DNA into host DNA
What is the function of gp120?	gp120 mediates binding to receptors on host cell surfaces.
What is the function of gp41?	gp41 mediates fusion of the virus to the cell membrane.
Why has it been difficult to produce effective vaccines targeting gp120?	The *env* gene mutates rapidly, resulting in many antigenic variants of gp120.

HIV

What are the main serotypes of HIV?

HIV-1 and HIV-2

What are the differences between HIV-1 and HIV-2?

HIV-1 is found worldwide while HIV-2 is found primarily in West Africa. HIV-2 causes less severe disease than HIV-1 and is less transmissible.

In addition to the three genes found in all retroviruses, what other genes are found in HIV and what do they encode?

tat gene—encodes tat, which enhances transcription of viral genes

rev gene—encodes rev, which facilitates transport of mRNA from nucleus to cytoplasm

nef gene—encodes nef, which represses synthesis of class I major histocompatibility complex (MHC) proteins, thus reducing the ability of cytotoxic T cells to kill infected cells

vif, *vpr*, and *vpu* genes—all accessory genes not required for viral replication

HIV binds primarily to what protein on a host cell?

CD4, which is bound by the gp120 envelope protein of HIV

On what type of cells' membrane is CD4 found?

Helper T cells, macrophages, and dendritic cells

What other receptor is necessary for HIV infection of a host cell?

Chemokine receptors CXCR4 (found on T cells) and CCR5 (found on macrophages)

What happens in people with homozygous mutations in the *CCR5* gene?

People with homozygous mutations are completely protected from HIV infection. Approximately 1% of people of Western European ancestry have the homozygous mutation.

What happens in people with heterozygous mutations in the *CCR5* gene?

Heterozygotes progress to disease more slowly. Approximately 10% to 15% of people of Western European ancestry have the heterozygous mutation.

How is HIV transmitted?

Sexual contact, transfer of infected blood, and perinatally

What are the three ways HIV is transmitted perinatally?

1. Across the placenta
2. At birth
3. Through breast milk

What has been shown to decrease the risk of perinatal HIV transmission?

Zidovudine (AZT) to pregnant mothers, cesarean delivery (if mother has high or unknown viral load), and avoiding breast-feeding

What is the rate of vertical transmission in untreated and treated (with AZT) seropositive pregnant mothers?

25% and 8%, respectively

Which has a lower infectious dose: HIV or HBV?

HBV has a lower infectious dose and thus is more efficiently transmitted.

What is the risk of being infected by HIV being stuck by a hollow bore needle from an HIV-positive patient?

Approximately 0.3%

Can HIV be transmitted via blood transfusions?

Yes. However, blood banks now routinely screen for HIV antibodies and p24 (which can detect HIV infection prior to the development of antibodies).

Does HIV affect cell-mediated or humoral immunity?

Cell-mediated immunity

Can HIV affect humoral immunity?

Yes. Abnormalities in B cells are seen in HIV-infected individuals, including polyclonal activation of B cells with resultant hyperimmunoglobulinemia and autoimmune disease such as thrombocytopenia.

What is the main immune response to HIV infection?

Cytotoxic T cells control spread of HIV in helper T cells. Some antibodies are produced against HIV, but appear to have little effect on curbing the infection.

Why do cytotoxic T cells fail to suppress HIV infection over time?

Cytotoxic T cells require activation by lymphokines released from helper T cells. As helper T cells die over time, the supply of lymphokines to activate cytotoxic T cells becomes insufficient.

How is HIV infection diagnosed? How many weeks after infection are antibodies formed?

Antibody detection by enzyme-linked immunosorbent assay (ELISA), followed by Western blot analysis. Antibodies form 3 to 4 weeks after infection.

Up to what age are ELISA and Western blot analysis unreliable for infants born to seropositive mothers? Why?

These infants are seropositive at birth regardless of infection status due to transplacental passage of maternal anti-HIV antibodies, which remain detectable up to *18 months of age.*

What tests can be used to detect HIV infection before antibody formation and in infants younger than 18 months born to seropositive mothers?

p24 antigen test, polymerase chain reaction (PCR) assay for HIV RNA, viral culture (not common)

What are the three stages of HIV infection?

1. Early acute stage
2. Middle latent stage
3. Late immunodeficient stage

What are signs and symptoms of early acute HIV infection?

Fever, lethargy, sore throat, generalized lymphadenopathy (similar to the clinical picture for infectious mononucleosis) along with maculopapular rash. These symptoms usually self-resolve in 2 weeks.

What percentage of individuals experience symptoms during the acute infection?

Up to 85%. Approximately 15% are asymptomatic after the initial infection.

What laboratory test is used to monitor response to treatment?

Viral load (copies of viral RNA/mL of plasma) and CD4 count

Does the middle latent stage refer to viral latency, clinical latency, or both?

Clinical latency only. The virus still replicates during the latent stage.

Where is the virus replicating during the latency stage?

Within the lymph nodes. Patients typically have low or absent viremia during the latent stage because the virus is sequestered within lymph nodes.

What is ARC?

AIDS-related complex. A syndrome of persistent fevers, fatigue, weight loss, and lymphadenopathy during the latent stage

When does an HIV-infected individual have AIDS?

When CD4 count drops below 200 cells/mL or after the presence of an AIDS-defining illness.

What are the two most common AIDS-defining malignancies?

1. Kaposi sarcoma
2. Lymphoma

What are common bacterial AIDS-defining infections?

Mycobacterium avium complex (MAC), *Mycobacterium tuberculosis, Streptococcus pneumoniae,* and *Salmonella*

Mnemonic: two are *Mycobacterium*; two affect sickle cell patients (*S. pneumoniae, Salmonella*).

What are common viral AIDS-defining infections?

Cytomegalovirus (CMV), JC virus, Epstein-Barr virus, Herpes simplex virus (1 and 2), and **Human** herpes virus 8 (associated with Kaposi sarcoma)

Mnemonic: Can **J**ust **E**asily **H**arm **Human**s

What are common fungal AIDS-defining infections?

*Candida, Coccidioides, **Crypt**ococcus,* and *Histoplasma*

Mnemonic: Can **C**ause **Crypt**ic **H**armful infections

What are common fungal and parasitic AIDS-defining infections?

Pneumocystis jiroveci (formerly *Pneumocystis carinii*), *Cryptosporidium, Toxoplasma gondii,* and *Isospora*

Mnemonic: Parasites **C**ause **T**errible **I**nfections.

For what infections should a HIV-infected individual should receive prophylaxis medication when CD4 count drops below 200 cells/mL?

Pneumocystis jiroveci pneumonia with trimethoprim-sulfamethoxazole (TMP-SMX). Note that the acronym PCP is maintained as an abbreviation for *Pneumocystis* pneumonia (*P. carinii* is now known to be a distinct species found in rats while *P. jiroveci* is a species found only in humans).

For what additional infections should n HIV-infected individual receive prophylaxis medication when CD4 count drops below 100 cells/mL?

Toxoplasma if seropositive with trimethoprim-sulfamethoxazole

For what additional infections an HIV-infected individual should receive prophylaxis medication when CD4 count drops below 50 cells/mL?

Mycobacterium avium complex with azithromycin, CMV if seropositive with ganciclovir, and *Histoplasma* if from an endemic area or with high-risk occupational exposure

What vaccines should all HIV individuals receive?

Influenza, pneumococcal, HBV (if antihepatitis B core antigen negative [anti-HBcAg negative]), hepatitis A virus (HAV) (if anti-HAV negative)

TREATMENT OF HIV

When is antiretroviral treatment begun for an HIV-infected individual?

Treatment is recommended for HIV-positive patients.

What are the classes of anti-HIV drugs?

1. Nucleoside reverse-transcriptase inhibitors (NRTIs)
2. Nonnucleoside reverse-transcriptase inhibitors (NNRTIs)
3. Protease inhibitors (PIs)
4. Integrase inhibitors (INSTIs)
5. Fusion inhibitors (FIs)
6. Chemokine receptor antagonists (CCR5 antagonists)
7. CD4- directed postattachment inhibitors

How do NRTIs work?

Competitive binding to reverse transcriptase after activation via phosphorylation by host enzymes

What are some examples of NRTIs?

Zidovudine (AZT), lamivudine (3TC), didanosine (ddI), zalcitabine (ddC), stavudine (d4T) (**-ine**), and abacavir

How do NNRTIs work?

Binds to reverse transcriptase at site separate from active site targeted by NRTIs and inhibits reverse transcriptase from forming DNA

What are some examples of NNRTIs?

Ne**vir**apine, efa**vir**enz, dela**vir**dine

What are some side effects of NNRTIs?

Rash, Steven Johnson syndrome, hepatotoxicity, vivid dreams, CNS symptoms

Which NNRTIs are teratogenic?

Delavirdine, efavirenz

How do PIs work?

Competitively inhibits cleavage of Gag-Pol polyproteins resulting in immature virions that are not infectious.

What are some examples of PIs?

Indinavir, saquinavir, ritonavir, and nelfinavir

Mnemonic: Protease inhibitors are Never Alone against the **VIR**us (-**NAVIR**).

Can a patient who develops resistance to an NRTI be switched to another NRTI?

Yes

Can a patient who develops resistance to a PI be switched to another PI?

No, resistance to one PI indicates resistance to all PIs.

What is a *buffalo hump*?

Fat deposition in the back of the neck associated with PI use. Also seen in Cushing syndrome.

How do integrase inhibitors (INSTIs) work?

Prevents integration of HIV DNA into host cell DNA

How do fusion inhibitors (FIs) work?

Binds to envelope glycoprotein 41 (gp41) of HIV to prevent viral

How do chemokine receptor antagonists (CCR5 antagonists) work?

HIV uses CD4 receptors with a coreceptor, chemokine coreceptor 5 (CCR5) or CXC chemokine coreceptor 4 (CXCR4). CCR5 antagonists only block HIV entry if the virus is the specific type that uses CCR5 (termed R5 viruses).

HTLV

What two diseases are associated with HTLV-1 infection?

1. Adult T-cell leukemia/lymphoma (ATLL)
2. HTLV-associated myelopathy (HAM). HTLV is an abbreviation for human T-cell leukemia virus or human T-cell lymphotropic virus.

What is HAM also known as?

Tropical spastic paraparesis or chronic progressive myelopathy

What is HAM? What are the clinical features of HAM?

A demyelinating disease of the brain and motor neurons of the spinal cord, thought to be caused by an autoimmune reaction resulting in gait disturbance, weakness of lower limbs, low back pain, primarily in women of middle age

What are the clinical features of HTLV-1–associated adult T-cell leukemia/lymphoma?

Lymphadenopathy, hepatosplenomegaly, lytic bone lesions, skin lesions, reduced cell-mediate immunity, hypercalcemia

What types of T cells does HTLV-1 infect?

CD4 helper T cells

To what genes in HIV are the *tax* and *rex* genes of HTLV-1 similar in function?

tat and *rev* genes of HIV

How is HTLV-1 different from other oncogenic viruses?	Its genome does not contain oncogenes and does not integrate into sites near cellular oncogenes.
How does HTLV-1 promote oncogenesis?	The tax protein promotes the synthesis of interleukin 2 (IL-2), leading to uncontrolled T-cell growth and eventual malignant transformation of the cell.
How is HTLV-1 typically transmitted?	Intravenous drug use, sexual contact, or breast-feeding.
Which areas have an endemic infection of HTLV-1?	Caribbean region, eastern South America, western Africa, and southern Japan
What is the treatment of HTLV-1 infection?	There are no therapies to treat the infection, though patients do undergo chemotherapy for HTLV-associated lymphoma/leukemia
What diseases are associated with HTLV-2?	HTLV-2 is closely related to HTLV-1 and is rarely associated with HAM.

CLINICAL VIGNETTES

A human immunodeficiency virus (HIV)-positive patient with a CD4 count of 100 cells/mm^3 was found to have a brain abscess that contained a gram-positive organism that stains weakly acid-fast. What is the organism and what is the treatment for choice?

Nocardia asteroides, trimethoprim-sulfamethoxazole (TMP-SMX)

A 25-year-old man with a history of AIDS presents with red purple plaques on his foot and the tip of his nose. The lesions are caused by a viral infection. Describe the morphology and genome causal organism:

The description earlier is that of Kaposi sarcoma, which is caused by human herpesvirus 8, an enveloped, icosahedral capsid with double-stranded linear DNA genome.

An HIV-positive patient, with a recent history of unprotected sex, presents with nonpruritic skin eruption consisting of numerous firm, painless 2- to 5-mm umbilicated nodules on his arms, trunk, and genital area. His palms and soles are spared. Microscopic examination of material expressed from the lesions reveals large cytoplasmic inclusions. What are the causative organism and clinical diagnosis? Describe the morphology of the causative organism:

Poxvirus causing molluscum contagiosum. Enveloped, complex structure, double-stranded DNA virus

A young man with AIDS presents with progressive shortness of breath, a dry painful cough, and a low-grade fever over weeks. He is hypoxic and his chest x-ray shows bilateral interstitial infiltrates. You obtain lung tissue to pursue your suspected diagnosis. What are you looking for under the microscope?

Cysts containing oval bodies (merozoites) for possible *Pneumocystis* pneumonia (PCP). *Pneumocystis* abundant on methenamine-silver stain, Giemsa stain, or fluorescent-antibody stain

CHAPTER 26

Remaining DNA Viruses

SMALLPOX VIRUS

Smallpox virus (first disease to be completely eradicated) is from which virus family?

Poxvirus

Describe the morphology and genome of poxviruses:

Enveloped, complex capsid with double-stranded linear DNA genome. Smallpox is actually the largest virus.

Mnemonic: Smallpox is actually LARGEpox.

How is smallpox transmitted?

Respiratory droplets, direct contact from fomite objects (i.e., inanimate objects that can transmit the disease)

What kind of vaccine is the smallpox vaccine?

Live attenuated

ADENOVIRUSES

What diseases do adenoviruses cause?

Pharyngitis, pneumonia, conjunctivitis ("pink eye"), the common cold, gastroenteritis, and hemorrhagic cystitis

Describe the morphology and genome of adenoviruses:

Nonenveloped, icosahedral capsid with double-stranded linear DNA genome

What cell type does adenovirus infect?	Mucosal epithelium throughout the body (i.e., respiratory tract, gastrointestinal tract, conjunctiva, and bladder epithelium). Note that different serotypes have predilections for what they infect (e.g., serotypes 8 and 19 cause epidemic keratoconjunctivitis).
What are the three routes of transmission for adenoviruses? Which one is the most common?	Respiratory aerosol, fecal-oral route, and iatrogenic inoculation of conjunctiva. Fecal-oral is the most common.
Keeping the above routes of transmission in mind, what populations are most at risk for outbreaks of infection?	Groups of people in close-living conditions (e.g., military, dormitories)
How is the virus spread within the host itself?	By cell lysis. After a sufficient number of virions assemble, the cell lyses, releasing the virus into the extracellular space

What are the symptoms associated with the following organ systems affected by adenovirus?

Ocular	Conjunctivitis
Upper respiratory system	Fever, sore throat, coryza
Lower respiratory system	Bronchitis, atypical pneumonia
Urinary tract	Hemorrhagic cystitis dysuria
GI	Nonbloody diarrhea in children younger than 2 years

Of the above organ systems, which two are most commonly simultaneously involved?	1. Conjunctiva 2. Upper respiratory system
How are adenovirus infections typically diagnosed?	Fourfold increase in antibody titer

HUMAN PAPILLOMAVIRUS

What diseases are caused by human papillomavirus (HPV)?

Plantar warts, genital warts, and cervical cancer

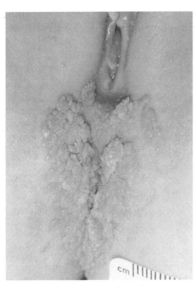

Figure 26.1   Anogenital warts caused by HPV. (*With permission from Fauci AS, Braunwald E, Kasper DL, et al.* Harrison's Principles of Internal Medicine. *17th ed. McGraw-Hill, NY; 2008.*)

What is the most common sexually transmitted disease (STD)?

HPV is probably by far the most common STD.

Describe the morphology and genome of HPV:

Nonenveloped, icosahedral capsid with double-stranded circular DNA genome

What are the names of the two genes that play a role in carcinogenesis?

1. *E6*
2. *E7*

E6 and E7 are carcinogenic by inactivating two tumor suppressor genes. What are two tumor suppressor genes that E6 and E7 inactivate, respectively?

1. E6 inactivates p53 gene.
2. E7 inactivates Rb gene.

Mnemonic: 6 is before 7 and P is before R (E6 = p53, E7 = Rb).

Which HPV serotypes predispose to cervical cancer?

HPV serotypes 16 and 18 account for roughly 70% of the serotypes that cause cervical cancer. Serotypes 31 and 33 are also considered high risk.

Why is HPV serotype 16 more likely to cause cancer than other serotypes?	HPV serotype 16 encodes an E6 and E7 protein that inhibits p53/Rb extremely effectively.
Besides cervical cancer, what other types of cancer does HPV cause?	Penile and anal cancers (might be the leading cause of anal cancer in homosexual men)
How is HPV transmitted?	Genital contact, skin-to-skin contact. Note that condoms do not prevent spread of HPV.
Pathology Correlate: What is the histologic hallmark of HPV infection?	Koilocytes with nuclear atypia and delayed maturation
Which HPV serotypes cause condylomata acuminate (genital warts)?	HPV serotypes 4 through 11
How are HPV infections diagnosed?	Acetic acid on HPV-associated lesions develops a characteristic acetowhite appearance, cytology for the presence of koilocytes, and molecular detection of HPV DNA.
What are some treatment options for HPV warts?	Topical removal, salicylic acid, podophyllin, α-interferon, and liquid nitrogen
What is the treatment of severe HPV infection?	Cidofovir (drug commonly used for CMV retinitis)
Is there an HPV vaccine?	Yes. There are three versions of the vaccine and they all cover the primary serotypes (16 and 18) that cause cancer.

PARVOVIRUS

What diseases does parvovirus B19 cause?	Erythema infectiosum (fifth disease), aplastic anemia, arthritis, and nonimmune hydrops fetalis **Mnemonic: PAR**vo (**P**regnancy-related hydrops fetalis, **A**plastic anemia/arthritis, **R**ash-Erythema infectiosum)
Describe the morphology and genome of parvovirus B19:	Small, nonenveloped, icosahedral capsid with single-stranded DNA genome

During which phase of the cellular cycle does parvovirus B19 virus replicate?

Only in the S phase when cellular DNA polymerase is present as the virus is dependent on cellular DNA polymerase

What are the primary means of viral transmission?

Respiratory aerosol and transplacental

How common is exposure to the virus in the United States?

Very common. Approximately 50% of people in the United States have antibodies to parvovirus B19.

What are the two main cell types infected by parvovirus?

1. RBC precursors in the bone marrow
2. Endothelial cells in the blood vessels

Considering that RBC precursors are one of the main cell types infected by parvovirus B19, what kind of disease can result from infection with the virus in susceptible individuals?

Aplastic anemia

What population is susceptible to transient aplastic crises characterized by severe weakness, lethargy, and undetectable peripheral reticulocytes?

Patients with sickle cell disease, hereditary spherocytosis, or baseline anemia (e.g., iron deficiency)

What condition are immunocompromised patients more likely to develop from parvovirus B19?

Chronic anemia (i.e., anemia may persist until immune function returns)

Parvovirus B19 can also cause disease, usually in children, with symptoms of bright red *slapped cheeks* rash, low-grade fever, sore throat, and coryza. What is the name of this disease?

Erythema infectiosum (slapped cheek syndrome) or fifth disease (it is the fifth disease discovered to cause a maculopapular rash in children)

What are the other diseases that cause a maculopapular rash in children?

Measles (first disease), scarlet fever from *Streptococcus pyogenes* (second disease), rubella (third disease), Duke disease from enteroviruses, echoviruses, and coxsackieviruses (fourth disease), and roseola from HHV6 (sixth disease)

What fetal outcome is associated with the infection of parvovirus during the first trimester of pregnancy?

Fetal death

What is the outcome if the infection occurs during the second trimester?

Hydrops fetalis (i.e., massive edema of the child characterized by skin edema, pleural effusions, polyhydramnios, ascites, and pericardial effusions)

How about infection during the third trimester?

Not clinically significant

CLINICAL VIGNETTE

On routine gynecologic examination, a woman with a history of unprotected sex has a few small, raised flat lesions on the cervix and genital warts on her vulva (condylomata acuminata). Micropathology reveals severe cervical dysplasia. What is the likely causative organism?

Human papillomavirus (HPV). Note that cervical dysplasia and condylomata acuminata are caused by different strains of HPV.

CHAPTER 27

Remaining RNA Viruses

RHABDOVIRUS

Describe the morphology and genome of rhabdoviruses. How is the shape of rhabdoviruses unique?	Enveloped, helical capsid with single-stranded negative-polarity RNA genome. The virus has a bullet-like shape.
How are rhabdoviruses transmitted to humans?	Via animal bites (e.g., dogs, skunks, raccoons, foxes, and bats are the most common reservoirs)
What is the mechanism by which the rhabdovirus infects the host?	The virus initially replicates at the bite site for several days to months. It then travels retrograde up the nervous system, eventually infecting neurons of the brain stem and brain.
Pathology Correlate: How is rabies infection diagnosed histologically? In what cells are they often seen?	Negri bodies, which are cytoplasmic inclusions that can be seen in the cytoplasm of infected neurons (especially hippocampal cells and Purkinje cells of the cerebellum)
What are the symptoms of rabies infection?	First a general prodrome of fever, fatigue, and headache, along with pain around the healed wound site followed by neurological sequelae characterized by agitation, confusion, and seizures. Cranial nerve dysfunction develops causing painful contraction of the pharyngeal muscles upon swallowing liquids (hydrophobia) or saliva (causing foaming of the mouth). Death occurs 1 to 2 weeks after onset of symptoms due to respiratory dysfunction.

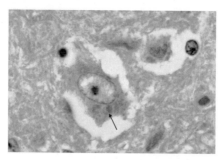

Figure 27.1 Rabies virus (note arrow on Negri body). (*With permission from Levinson WE.* Review of Medical Microbiology and Immunology. *10th ed. New York, NY: McGraw-Hill; 2008.*)

How is the rabies vaccine administered?

The vaccine is given preexposure to individuals in high-risk groups. It can also be administered postexposure with antirabies immune globulin during the long incubation period.

FILOVIRUS

Describe the morphology and genome of filoviruses:

Enveloped, helical capsid with nonsegmented, single-stranded, negative-polarity RNA genome

What are the two filoviruses that cause human disease? What are their respective reservoirs?

1. Marburg virus (monkey reservoir)
2. Ebola virus (unknown reservoir, although some evidence suggests that bats are the reservoir)

Both viruses cause hemorrhagic fever through epidemic cycles.

How are Ebola and Marburg viruses transmitted?

Via direct contact with bodily fluid of an infected individual

What is the pathogenesis of these diseases?

Viremia leading to flu-like symptoms and soon organ failure with focal necrosis and internal hemorrhage. Death within 1 to 2 weeks from septic shock/multiple-organ failure

| What is the mortality rate of these diseases? | 70% to 90% mortality for Ebola virus and 80% to 90% mortality for Marburg virus. No treatment or vaccine exists for either infection. |

ARENAVIRUS

What is the medically significant arenavirus?	Lassa virus that causes Lassa fever, a form of hemorrhagic fever
Describe the morphology and genome of arenaviruses:	Enveloped, helical capsid with two nonidentical, single-stranded, negative-polarity RNA segments
What is the reservoir of the Lassa virus and how is it transmitted?	Rodent reservoir. Transmitted to humans via contamination of food or water by rodent urine. Secondary transmission then occurs from person to person through bodily fluids.
What is the pathogenesis of this disease?	Infection causes viremia leading to hemorrhagic fever and eventually hemorrhagic shock. Often difficult to distinguish from other hemorrhagic fevers such as Ebola
What is the treatment of Lassa fever?	Early administration of ribavirin reduces mortality. Hyperimmune serum from recovered patients partially decreases mortality.

REOVIRUS

What are the medically significant reoviruses?	Rotavirus and coltivirus
Describe the morphology and genome of reoviruses:	Nonenveloped, icosahedral capsid with segmented, double-stranded RNA. They are the only medically significant double-stranded RNA viruses.
How is rotavirus transmitted?	Via fecal-oral route

What is the pathogenesis of rotavirus infection and how does it lead to symptoms?

This virus initially infects and replicates in the mucosal cells of the proximal small intestine. It lyses these cells, thereby damaging the intestinal transport mechanisms. This leads to the loss of minerals, electrolytes, and water through vomit and watery diarrhea. The diarrhea is nonbloody.

What is the epidemiological significance of rotavirus?

Most common worldwide cause of infectious diarrhea in infants and young children (>1 million infant deaths annually). Norwalk virus is the most common cause in adults and older children.

Is there a vaccine for rotavirus? What is a classic complication of the vaccine?

Yes. It is a live-attenuated vaccine taken orally. Classically the vaccine has been associated with intussusception.

How is coltivirus transmitted?

Coltivirus is carried in rodents and transmitted via a wood-tick vector. The disease is endemic to the Rocky Mountains and infects hikers and campers.

What is the pathogenesis of coltivirus infection?

Infection leads to viremia and multiorgan lesions causing fever, headache, retro-orbital pain, and myalgia. Pancytopenia may result from bone marrow involvement.

NORWALK VIRUS

Of which family of viruses is Norwalk virus, also known as norovirus, a member?

Calicivirus

Describe the morphology and genome of Norwalk viruses:

Nonenveloped, icosahedral capsid with nonsegmented, single-stranded, positive-polarity RNA genome

What is the pathogenesis of Norwalk virus infection?

It is transmitted fecal-orally and causes vomiting and nonbloody diarrhea through a similar mechanism to rotavirus. Symptoms typically last only 1 to 2 days.

What is the epidemiological significance of Norwalk virus infection?

It is the most common worldwide cause of infectious diarrhea in adults and older children. Classic exam presentation of diarrheal illness on a cruise ship.

RHINOVIRUS AND CORONAVIRUS

Describe the morphology of coronaviruses and rhinoviruses:

Both are nonsegmented, single-stranded, positive-polarity RNA viruses. Coronavirus is enveloped with a helical capsid. Rhinovirus is nonenveloped with an icosahedral capsid.

What do rhinovirus and coronavirus commonly cause?

They both cause the common cold. Rhinovirus is the most common cause (50%) and coronavirus is the second most common (20%).

What other viruses cause the common cold?

Adenovirus, influenza C virus, and coxsackievirus

What times of year do most coronavirus and rhinovirus infections occur?

Coronavirus infections occur in winter/early spring. Rhinovirus infections occur in summer, fall, and early winter.

Does rhinovirus cause lower respiratory tract infections? Why or why not?

No. Rhinoviruses replicate better at 33°C than at the body temperatures of 37°C. Thus, it preferentially infects the cooler areas of the body (nose and upper airways).

What is the pathogenesis of rhinovirus infection?

The virus binds intercellular adhesion molecule 1 (ICAM-1) on the surface of upper respiratory tract epithelial cells causing local release of cytokines and upregulation of ICAM-1 expression in the epithelial cells. The release of cytokines causes the symptoms of the cold and the increase of ICAM-1 expression promotes local propagation of the infection.

What treatments are available for these infections?

Supportive treatment with nonsteroidal anti-inflammatory drugs (NSAIDs), acetaminophen, antihistamines, and decongestants

What other strain of coronavirus causes disease in humans?

The SARS (severe acute respiratory syndrome) virus, which caused an outbreak of severe respiratory infection in parts of Asia in 2003

POLIOVIRUS, COXSACKIEVIRUS, AND ECHOVIRUS

Poliovirus, coxsackievirus, and echovirus known as enteroviruses are all members of which viral family?

Picornavirus family. Hepatitis A and rhinovirus are also part of the picornavirus family.

Describe the morphology and genome of picornaviruses:

Nonenveloped, icosahedral capsid with nonsegmented, single-stranded, positive-polarity RNA genome

How are enteroviruses uniquely adapted to infections of the enteric tract?

The enteroviruses replicate optimally at 37°C, are not inactivated under acidic conditions, and are nonenveloped for greater stability.

How are enteroviruses typically transmitted?

Fecal-oral. Coxsackievirus can also be transmitted through aerosol.

What is the shared pathogenesis of all enterovirus infections?

The viral capsid protein binds to a receptor on the oral pharynx or small intestine epithelium. It replicates in the submucosal lymphoid tissues of these areas and then enters the bloodstream to cause a transient viremia.

What is the specific pathogenesis of poliovirus infection?

Following viremia, it spreads to the central nervous system (CNS) via blood or retrograde transport in peripheral nerves. It infects and lyses motor neurons of the anterior horn of the spinal cord causing denervation of various muscle groups.

What are the clinical symptoms of poliovirus infection?

90% to 95% of infected individuals are asymptomatic. A small percentage get abortive poliomyelitis (fever, headache, sore throat, nausea/vomiting). Another small percentage get nonparalytic poliomyelitis, with clinical signs of aseptic meningitis. Less than 1% of infected patients will develop paralytic poliomyelitis. Flaccid paralysis occurs if distal muscles are involved, but brain-stem involvement can lead to life-threatening respiratory paralysis.

How are poliovirus infections treated?

Symptomatic support. But two vaccines are available, the Salk (inactivated poliovirus vaccine [IPV]) and the Sabin (oral poliovirus vaccine live [OPV]).

How does the Salk (IPV) vaccine work?

Salk is a killed virus vaccine administered subcutaneously and provokes an immunoglobulin G (IgG) response to protect against future viremia. The inactivated virus cannot revert to virulence, which makes it the preferential choice for use in immunocompromised individuals.

How does the Sabin vaccine work?

Sabin is a live-attenuated virus vaccine administered orally and generates IgA mucosal immunity in addition to systemic IgG immunity. The attenuated virus can spread to contacts from fecal oral route resulting in immunity in these individuals. Strain can also revert to a virulent form.

How many types of coxsackievirus are there? How are they classified?

There are two types of coxsackievirus: A and B. Classification is based on their pathogenicity in mice.

What are the top three viral causes of aseptic meningitis?

1. Coxsackievirus
2. Echovirus
3. Mumps virus

What symptoms are common to both types A and B?

Both types can cause aseptic meningitis and paralysis through involvement of the meninges and anterior horn motor neurons. They can also cause upper respiratory tract infection by dissemination through the bloodstream.

What are the pathogenesis and clinical symptoms specific to coxsackievirus A?

Type A has a predilection for skin and mucosal membranes and causes herpangina (fever, sore throat, and tender red vesicles on the back of the throat) and hand-foot-mouth disease (vesicular rash on the hands and feet and ulcerations in the mouth).

What are the pathogenesis and clinical symptoms specific to coxsackievirus B?

Type B has a predilection for the heart and pleural surfaces and causes pleurodynia (fever, headache, and severe chest pain on breathing due to pleural infection), myocarditis (50% of all viral cases), and pericarditis (chest pain, arrhythmias, cardiomyopathy, or heart failure). Pancreatic damage possibly leading to juvenile diabetes may also occur.

What treatment is available for coxsackievirus infections?

There are no treatments or vaccines available.

What are the symptoms of echovirus infection?

Aseptic meningitis (second leading cause), upper respiratory infections, fever with or without rash, infantile diarrhea, and hemorrhagic conjunctivitis

CHAPTER 28

Prions

What is an infectious prion?	A modified form of a normal nervous system structural protein
What is the normal prion protein and where in the human genome is it located?	The normal prion protein is associated with the cell membrane and is coded for chromosome 20 of the human genome.
How are prions unique from other types of infectious agents?	They are the only class of infectious agent that does not contain nucleic acids, RNA, or DNA (i.e., they are purely protein).
How are prion-related diseases acquired?	Either by sporadic mutation (85%), inheritance of a mutated gene (15%), or through an infectious mechanism
What is the pathological mechanism by which infectious prions cause disease?	A normal prion (PrP^c) undergoes a structural change to become an abnormal prion protein (PrP^{sc}). PrP^{sc} induces other PrP^c generating large numbers of PrP^{sc}.
What is the major structural difference between PrP^c and PrP^{sc}?	PrP^c has α-helices while PrP^{sc} has β-pleated sheets.
Why are infectious prions harder to sterilize than viruses or bacteria?	Prions are far more resistant to inactivation by ultraviolet light and heat than are viruses and bacteria. Additionally, prions are very resistant to formaldehyde and nucleases (prions have no nucleic acid).
What is unique about the body's immune response to a prion infection?	Prion protein is the product of a normal cellular gene, so no immune response is generated.

Pathology Correlate: Which part of the brain tissue is most commonly affected by prion-related disease and what is the histological appearance of prion-infected brain tissue?

Gray matter. Vacuoles within the brain stroma and cell bodies of the gray matter result in spongiform change. The disorder is called a spongiform encephalopathy.

What are the four human prion diseases that have been identified so far?

1. Creutzfeldt-Jakob disease (human *mad cow disease*)
2. Kuru
3. Gerstmann-Sträussler-Scheinker disease
4. Fatal familial insomnia

How are infectious prions transmitted?

Contaminated neural tissue is inoculated/ingested. Iatrogenic cases of Creutzfeldt-Jakob disease have been associated with contaminated neurosurgical instruments, cadaveric dural grafts, corneal transplants, and human pituitary extracts. No evidence of blood transmission has been shown.

What are the clinical features shared by all prion diseases?

Psychiatric symptoms, rapidly progressing dementia, cerebellar symptoms (ataxia, startle myoclonus). All of these diseases are completely fatal, as there is no treatment available.

List some diagnostic studies and classically findings suggestive of prion diseases?

Lumbar puncture showing 14-3-3 protein.

EEG showing "periodic sharp wave complexes"

T2 MRI showing hyperintensity of caudate and putamen

Histology of spongiform cortex (generally postmortem) showing large intracellular vacuoles

SECTION V

Mycology

CHAPTER 29

General Principles of Mycology

How are fungi different from bacteria?

Fungi are eukaryotic with a true nucleus, 80S ribosomes, mitochondria, and endoplasmic reticulum. Bacteria are prokaryotic with no true nucleus, 70S ribosomes, no mitochondria, and no endoplasmic reticulum.

Describe the cell membrane and cell wall of fungi:

Cell membrane contains ergosterol and cell wall contains chitin, glucan, and mannan. All have been utilized as targets for antifungal drugs.

Are fungi heterotrophic (require carbon) or autotrophic (produce carbon)?

Heterotrophic. They can be parasitic (obtain carbon off another living organism), saprophytic (obtain carbon from dead organic material), or mutualistic (obtain carbon off another living organism in a symbiotic relationship).

What is the difference between molds and yeasts?

Yeasts are single-celled and reproduced by budding. Molds have hyphae, which are filamentous units, and grow by branching.

What is the difference between septate hyphae and nonseptate hyphae?

Septate hyphae have clear cross walls and fairly regular width. Nonseptate hyphae have no cross walls and irregular width.

What is a dimorphic fungus? Name the medically important dimorphic fungi:

A dimorphic fungus can exist as either a yeast or mold form, depending on its environment "Mold in the cold, yeast in the heat." Medically important dimorphic fungi include *Histoplasma*, *Blastomyces*, *Coccidioides*, and *Sporothrix*.

What are conidia?

Specialized nonmotile structure with asexual spores formed from an extension of the hyphal wall. Although fungi can also have sexual sporulation, asexual sporulation is more common in medically important fungi.

How are fungal infections typically classified?

By body location (i.e., cutaneous, subcutaneous, or systemic)

What is meant by opportunistic fungal infections?

Another category of fungal infection that occurs in immunosuppressed patients (e.g., human immunodeficiency virus [HIV], transplant patients)

How are fungal infections diagnosed?

Direct microscopic examination, culture of the organism, serologic tests, or DNA probes

Describe some common stains used to visualize fungi:

Potassium hydroxide (KOH) wet mount visualizes most hyphae and yeast by lysing cell membranes. Fungi remain unaffected due to cell wall; silver stain for *Pneumocystis jiroveci*; India ink stain of cerebrospinal fluid (CSF) is confirmatory for *Cryptococcus neoformans* meningitis.

What is the most common culture media used to culture fungi? Why?

Sabouraud agar. Low pH inhibits bacterial growth (antibiotics are sometimes added).

CHAPTER 30

Cutaneous and Subcutaneous Mycoses

CUTANEOUS MYCOSES

What are some common dermatophytes?	Microsporum, trichophyton, epidermophyton
What is tinea capitis?	Fungal scalp infection
What is tinea pedis?	Athlete's foot (i.e., fungal infection between toes and on soles of feet)
What is tinea corporis?	Ringworm of smooth skin
What is tinea cruris?	Jock itch (i.e., fungal infection of groin and perineal areas)
What is tinea unguium (onychomycosis)?	Fungal infection of the nails
What area of the skin do dermatophytes (fungi that infect skin/hair/nails) infect?	Nonviable keratinized layers
What chemical is added to a skin scraping to identify dermatophytes?	10% to 20% potassium hydroxide (KOH) solution. It lyses cell membranes so human skin cells are disrupted but fungi remain unaffected because they are protected by a cell wall.
What is Wood lamp?	365-nm wavelength ultraviolet (UV) light used to identify dermatophytoses

What culture medium is used for dermatophytes?

Sabouraud agar. Selects for fungi in skin, hair, and nails that are likely to be contaminated with bacteria

What is the most common cause of diaper rash?

Candida albicans

What is the most common form of tinea capitis in the United States?

Black dot tinea capitis. Patchy hair loss, common in pediatric patients, characterized by black dots in the scalp where the hair breaks. Most commonly caused by *Trichophyton tonsurans* and the alopecia may remain permanent if not treated

What is the treatment of choice for tinea capitis?

Griseofulvin (drug of choice), terbinafine, or itraconazole. Topical treatment usually fails.

How is acute tinea pedis diagnosed?

Clinical picture of pruritic lesions often between toes following activity. Confirmation with KOH-treated scrapings showing characteristic branching hyphae and culture on Sabouraud agar

How is chronic tinea pedis diagnosed?

Clinical picture of a progressive, erythematous lesion extending from the interdigital spaces to the soles with a sharp demarcation between infected and normal regions. Confirmation with KOH-treated examination and culture

How is tinea pedis treated?

Interdigital tinea can be treated with topical creams (e.g., terbinafine, clotrimazole). More extensive or chronic infections may require oral therapy such as terbinafine or itraconazole.

What is the most common coinfection with onychomycosis (fungal nail infection)?

Tinea pedis. Usually with *Trichophyton rubrum*

What is the differential diagnosis of nail infections?

Onychomycosis, psoriasis, eczematous conditions, senile ischemia, and lichen planus

How is the diagnosis of onychomycosis made?

KOH scrapings, culture on Sabouraud agar, or periodic acid-Schiff (PAS)–stained nail specimens

What is the treatment of choice for onychomycosis?

Oral terbinafine or itraconazole. Fluconazole is also effective, but griseofulvin is not.

How is tinea corporis (ring worm) diagnosed?	Appears as a slightly raised circular lesion with an erythematous border on the body. Often seen in patients exposed to tinea capitis/pedis (parents of children with either disease). Underlying medical conditions should be suspected when very extensive.
How is tinea corporis treated?	Topical antifungal creams. Extensive cases can be treated with oral agents.
How is tinea cruris diagnosed?	Appears as a macular patch on the inner thighs and spreads centrifugally. Diagnosed with a KOH scraping and culture. Usually caused by *T. rubrum*. Tinea cruris must be differentiated from a dermal infection by *C. albicans*.
How is tinea cruris treated?	The area should be kept dry with powders to prevent recurrences. Topical antifungal creams or oral antifungal agent are effective for active infections.

SUBCUTANEOUS MYCOSES

Describe the morphology of *Sporothrix schenckii*:	Dimorphic yeast that is cigar-shaped in tissue
How is *Sporothrix* transmitted?	Traumatic implantation, usually a thorn puncture (rose gardener's disease)
How does *Sporothrix* present?	Ulcer with characteristic chain of swollen draining lymph nodes (ascending lymphangitis)
How is *Sporothrix* treated?	Itraconazole or potassium iodide

CLINICAL VIGNETTE

A 27-year-old gardener presents to a physician with an ulcer on his left forearm for 2 weeks. On physical examination, he has a small ulcer on his left arm and several nodules moving up toward his left shoulder. He is nonfebrile. What is the most likely causative agent and how is it diagnosed?

Sporothrix schenckii (rose gardener's disease) infects a thorn puncture site and then moves along draining lymphatics, producing nodules. It is diagnosed by visualizing cigar-shaped budding yeast forms on biopsy.

CHAPTER 31

Systemic Mycoses

Name the four endemic fungi considered to cause systemic infections in humans:	1. *Histoplasma* 2. *Coccidioides* 3. *Blastomyces* 4. *Paracoccidioides*
Are all systemic fungi dimorphic?	Yes. They can exist as either yeast or mold forms.
In what form do they appear at body temperature?	Around body temperature (37°C) they grow as yeast forms on blood agar. At 25°C they grow as mold forms with spores on Sabouraud agar.
How do the systemic fungi enter the body?	Through inhalation of fungal spores
Is there person-to-person spread of these diseases?	No. Only spores are infective and must be inhaled directly from soil or bird droppings.
Describe three types of infection that systemic mycoses are known to cause:	1. Asymptomatic/mild upper respiratory infection (URI): majority of cases. 2. Pneumonia: a mild pneumonia with fever, cough, and infiltrates seen on x-ray. Note that infections with these organisms can cause calcified granulomas. 3. Disseminated: rare, usually in immunocompromised patients. The fungus spreads hematogenously from the lungs causing granulomatous infections throughout the body.
Which one of the above four fungi is a facultative intracellular parasite known to infect reticuloendothelial cells?	*Histoplasma capsulatum*

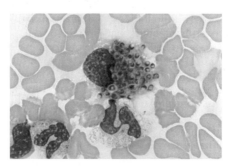

Figure 31.1   Macrophage containing histoplasmosis. (*With permission from Lichtman MA, Shafer MS, Felgar RE, Wang N.* Lichtman's Atlas of Hematology. *New York, NY: McGraw-Hill; 2007. Available at www.accessmedicine.com.*)

Histoplasma is often seen as oval budding yeast inside macrophages. What substances do the yeast produce that allows it to survive in the harsh environment of the phagolysosome?

The yeast produces alkaline substances such as bicarbonate and ammonia, which raise the pH of the phagolysosome thereby inactivating the degradative enzymes.

What areas of the country is *Histoplasma* endemic?

Eastern Great lakes, Ohio, Mississippi, and Missouri river valleys

In what season is histoplasmosis most common?

Summer

What animals are associated with *Histoplasma* infections?

Histoplasma is found in soil contaminated with bird or bat feces.

What activities put one at increased risk of contracting the disease?

Essentially any activities that expose one to bird and bat feces, including spelunking (cave exploring), cleaning chicken coops, or bulldozing starling roosts

Why is it useful to obtain peripheral blood smears in patients suspected with histoplasmosis infections?

Since *Histoplasma* circulates in reticuloendothelial system (RES) cells it can be seen in peripheral smears.

Describe the tissue form of the disease:

Small intracellular yeasts, which despite their name are not encapsulated.

In a patient with suspected histoplasmosis, what abnormality might be found on physical examination of the abdomen?

Hepatosplenomegaly since *Histoplasma* infects reticuloendothelial cells.

How is histoplasmosis treated?

Itraconazole and amphotericin B (reserved for moderate or severe infections)

In patients from the endemic areas, what radiographic findings suggest prior infection with *Histoplasma*?

Calcified granulomas in the spleen and lungs

Name the systemic fungus that is endemic in the southwestern United States whose environmental form resembles hyphae breaking up into arthroconidia found in desert sand:

Coccidioides immitis (valley fever)

Describe the morphology of the tissue form of *Coccidioides*:

Spherules with endospores

What skin rash is associated with *Coccidioides* infection?

Erythema nodosum. It is a skin disease characterized by tender red nodules found beneath the skin, usually on the shins, as well as fever, and joint pain. In cases of *Coccidioides* infections, it serves as a positive prognostic indicator suggesting an active cell-mediated immune response to the organism. However, other triggers can include drugs, pregnancy, malignancy, and inflammatory conditions.

Why is *Coccidioides* infection a concern in pregnant patients?

It has a tendency to disseminate in the third trimester of pregnancy.

What is the most important extrapulmonary site of dissemination?

Meninges

Describe the impact of race on the natural history of coccidioidomycoses:

Non-Caucasians have a higher rate of disseminated infection.

Name the systemic fungus whose tissue form resembles broad-based budding yeast:

Blastomyces dermatitidis

Which opportunistic fungus forms narrow-based budding yeast?

Cryptococcus neoformans

What is the endemic region associated with *Blastomyces*?

This fungus is found in the Great Lakes region, the Ohio, and Mississippi river valley, as well as the northeastern United States extending into Canada.

What is the environmental form of *Blastomyces*?

Hyphae with conidia

Whereas acute lesions with *Histoplasma* and *Coccidioides* often spontaneously resolve, with what medication are *Blastomyces* infections often treated?

Itraconazole. Amphotericin B may be used in severe disseminated cases.

Pharmacology Correlate: Name the serious side effects of amphotericin B that may limit its use in the clinical setting:

Renal toxicity (which is reversible if the drug is stopped), fevers and chills, anemia, hepatotoxicity, electrolyte imbalances, and phlebitis at the intravenous (IV) site

Which systemic fungus is endemic in rural Latin America?

Paracoccidioides brasiliensis, also known as South American blastomycosis, is found in the soil.

Which group of lymph nodes are affected by *P. brasilensis*?

Cervical chain lymphadenopathy

Describe the appearance of the yeast form of *Paracoccidioides*:

Paracoccidioides brasiliensis is thick-walled with multiple buds. Classically described as a "captain's wheel"

What bacterial infection may mimic systemic mycotic infection?

Mycobacterium tuberculosis can resemble systemic mycoses, as both are acquired through the respiratory route and cause asymptomatic to chronic lung infections, leaving granulomas, calcifications, and possibly cavitary lesions. Also, both can spread hematogenously, infecting distant body organs.

CLINICAL VIGNETTES

A 33-year-old man presents with an influenza-like illness with fever and cough, as well as a rash on the skin of his lower legs. While taking a thorough social history, you find out your patient is an avid runner who has recently gone running in the San Joaquin Valley. Given this important piece of history, what fungal infection should you consider on your differential diagnosis in addition to the common respiratory pathogens?

Coccidioides immitis is common in the desert area of the San Joaquin Valley. The above syndrome is commonly known as *valley fever* and often subsides without treatment.

A 28-year-old homosexual man presents to the physician with a headache and fever. His chart reveals multiple episodes of oral thrush and a prescription for trimethoprim-sulfamethoxazole (TMP-SMX) that the patient says he never filled because "I'm not sick." On examination, he has nuchal rigidity and his cerebrospinal fluid (CSF) shows low neutrophils, slightly low glucose, and normal protein. Gram stain is negative for bacteria, but does show some organisms. Follow-up stain with India ink shows small, round organisms surrounded by a clear halo. What is the causative organism and what is the next step in treatment?

Cryptococcus neoformans. Start intravenous (IV) amphotericin B plus 5-flucytosine

A 26-year-old man presents to your office with a cough and fever for 2 weeks. He complains that his cough might prevent him from going hiking with his friends next month. On further questioning, he admits to having been on a trip to Missouri about a month ago during which he explored a cave in which he found hundreds of bats. On physical examination, he has some rough rales in his right lower lung and a temperature of 101.2°F. Chest x-ray is normal. What is the most likely picture of this patient's transbronchial biopsy?

2- to 4-μm yeasts in macrophages indicative of *Histoplasma* infection upon staining with Wright stain

CHAPTER 32

Opportunistic Mycoses

What are the most common opportunistic mycoses?	Candidiasis caused by *Candida* Invasive aspergillosis caused by *Aspergillus* Cryptococcal meningitis caused by *Cryptococcus* Zygomycosis caused by *Mucor*, *Rhizopus*, and related species Interstitial pneumonia caused by *Pneumocystis jiroveci*
Describe the morphology of *Candida albicans*:	*Candida albicans* is an oval yeast with a single bud that forms pseudohyphae and true hyphae when it invades tissue. It exists simultaneously as mold and yeast form.
Where is *C. albicans* usually found?	*Candida albicans* is the most common cause of fungal infections in immuno-compromised patients. It is indigenous to the oropharyngeal membrane.
What diseases does *C. albicans* cause?	Mucocutaneous candidiasis (oral thrush, esophagitis, gastritis, and vaginitis). Up to 90% of human immunodeficiency virus (HIV) patients on highly active antiretro-viral therapy (HAART) will eventually develop mucocutaneous candidiasis. Seventy-five percent of all women will have at least one episode of vaginal candi-diasis. Systemic candidiasis with mortal-ity rates of 30% to 40%. *Candida* is also the leading cause of fungal endocarditis. **Mnemonic:** Treat w/**CVS** (a pharmacy) **M**eds (**C**arditis, **V**aginal, **S**ystemic, **M**ucocutaneous)

What sort of candida infections occur in neutropenic patients? Patients with T-cell dysfunction?

Systemic candidiasis with neutrophilic dysfunction. Localized candida infection with T-cell dysfunction

How is *C. albicans* diagnosed?

Potassium hydroxide (KOH) smear shows pseudohyphae, true hyphae, and budding yeasts.

What are some risk factors for vaginal candidiasis?

Diabetes mellitus, oral contraceptives, recent antibiotic use, immunodeficiency

How is *C. albicans* treated?

Nystatin for oral thrush, topical agents or fluconazole for localized infections, fluconazole or amphotericin for systemic infections

Describe the morphology of *Aspergillus*:

Monomorphic fungus with septate hyphae and dichotomous acute-angle branches

What diseases does *Aspergillus* cause?

Allergic bronchopulmonary aspergillosis, pulmonary aspergillosis (including aspergilloma, which is a fungus ball that develops in preexisting lung cavity), and invasive aspergillosis

What is allergic bronchopulmonary aspergillosis?

Complex hypersensitivity reaction to Aspergillus found almost exclusively in asthmatics and cystic fibrosis. Diagnosed using combination of radiographic (e.g., central bronchiectasis, high attenuation mucus) and clinical findings (e.g., asthma/CF, skin test/IgE levels).

What is the treatment for *Aspergillus*?

Voriconazole is essential element for most therapies with consideration for combination with an echinocandin (e.g., caspofungin) or amphotericin B.

Describe the morphology of *Cryptococcus neoformans*:

Encapsulated monomorphic fungus that forms a narrow-based bud

What is the most important disease caused by *Cryptococcus*?

Meningitis. Most common cause of meningitis in AIDS patients (up to 10% of all AIDS patients)

How are cryptococcal infections diagnosed?

Latex particle agglutination or India ink finding of *budding yeasts with capsules*

What radiographic finding can be found with cryptococcal meningoencephalitis?

Hydrocephalus. Also associated with increased opening pressure and may require shunt placement

Where is *Cryptococcus* found in the environment?

Bird (especially pigeon) droppings

What is the treatment of choice for cryptococcal meningoencephalitis?

Intravenous amphotericin B plus flucytosine for 2 weeks is the treatment of choice to sterilize the cerebrospinal fluid (CSF). Long-term maintenance therapy with oral fluconazole may be required for patients with underlying immunosuppression (e.g., AIDS, bone marrow transplant).

What genera of fungi most commonly cause zygomycosis (mucormycosis)?

Mucor or *Rhizopus*

What are the important risk factors for zygomycosis?

Diabetes, especially diabetic ketoacidosis (DKA), iron chelation therapy, neutropenia, immunosuppressive therapies

Why are diabetics and patients on iron chelation therapy more susceptible to zygomycosis?

Rhizopus has a ketone reductase that allows it to flourish in acidic high glucose environments such as DKA. Deferoxamine, an iron chelator, facilitates iron uptake by *Rhizopus* and thus encourages its growth.

What are the most common body sites for zygomycosis?

Rhinocerebral and thoracic (pulmonary)

***Mucor* and related species are angioinvasive and contribute to extensive tissue necrosis and infarction. What is the treatment for zygomycosis?**

Early surgical debridement with amphotericin B. Prognosis remains poor for both patients with rhinocerebral (mortality 25%–50%) and pulmonary (mortality up to 80%) infections.

What does *Rhizopus* look like on wet mount?

Large, nonseptate branching hyphae with greater than 90° angles

What is *Pneumocystis* pneumonia (PCP)?

Pneumocystis pneumonia, an AIDS-defining illness, caused by *P. jiroveci*. Up to 75% of AIDS patients eventually develop this disease. Note that older sources may still refer to *P. carinii*, but human disease is caused by *P. jiroveci*.

What type of cells do *P. jiroveci* attack?

Type I pneumocytes (large, thin cell involved in gas exchange and unable to replicate) causing excessive replication of type II pneumocytes (granular cell involved in surfactant secretion and capable of replication)

How is *P. jiroveci* diagnosed?

Fluorescent antibody, silver-stained cysts in bronchial alveolar lavage, or biopsy

At what CD4 count would you give prophylaxis for *P. jiroveci*?

When CD4<200

What is the treatment for *P. jiroveci* pneumonia?

Trimethoprim-sulfamethoxazole (TMP-SMX). If resistant or allergic, aerosolized pentamidine is an alternative.

CLINICAL VIGNETTE

A 34-year-old male immigrant presents to the physician with a cough and hemoptysis. Three years ago, his purified protein derivative (PPD) was positive and chest x-ray showed likely active tuberculosis. He was treated with isoniazid (INH) and rifampin and his symptoms abated. His chest x-ray reveals a blurry cavitating lesion in his right upper lobe and Ghon complex. What fungal infection is likely superimposed on his tuberculosis (TB)?

Aspergillus infection can insinuate itself into a cavitation from a prior illness and cause a *fungus ball* or *aspergilloma* in the space.

CHAPTER 33

Antifungal Drugs

What is the treatment for oral thrush?	Nystatin
What organisms is amphotericin B effective against?	Virtually every fungus. Some resistance has been reported among *Candida* species, but it remains the treatment of choice for virtually any life-threatening fungal infection.
What is the mechanism of action for amphotericin B? Which other antifungal has a similar mechanism?	Amphotericin B and nystatin binds to sterols (e.g., ergosterol) in fungal membranes and creates pores into the membrane leading to cell death.
What is lipid-based amphotericin B?	Amphotericin B is encased in a liposomal vesicle or lipid-based vesicle. It is associated with less toxicity.
To which family of antifungal drugs does fluconazole belong?	The triazole family. Other members are itraconazole and voriconazole.
What is the mechanism of action for the triazoles?	Inhibition of the enzyme cytochrome P450 14 α-demethylase, which converts lanosterol to ergosterol. It thus inhibits fungal steroid synthesis.
What are the major toxicities associated with fluconazole?	Although fluconazole is very well tolerated, associated side effects include gastrointestinal (GI) discomfort, rash, headache, liver toxicity (rarely), and alopecia (from long-term treatment).
Is fluconazole safe in pregnancy?	No. Fetal damage has been documented.
Do triazoles inhibit or induce the P450 system?	They inhibit the P450 enzymes. This can lead to interactions with warfarin, digitalis, cisapride, and so on.

What medication should not be administered with itraconazole?

Antacids or H2-inhibitors/proton pump inhibitors (PPIs). Itraconazole requires acidic pH for dissolution of capsules and should be given 2 hours before or after any antacids or H2-inhibitors/PPIs.

To which family of antifungal drugs Ketoconazole belong?

The imidazole family. Other members are clotrimazole and miconazole.

What is the mechanism of action of imidazoles?

Inhibition of the enzyme cytochrome P450 14α-demethylase, which converts lanosterol to ergosterol. Same mechanism as triazoles

What type of infections are the imidazoles used for?

Superficial infections. Ketoconazole is the treatment of choice for tinea versicolor and mucocutaneous candidiasis. Imidazole creams are used for yeast infections and various tinea infections. All have activity against *Candida* infections.

What toxicities are associated with ketoconazole?

Liver toxicity, GI upset, thrombocytopenia, and photophobia. Gynecomastia due to inhibition of estrogen metabolism also occurs.

Is ketoconazole an inhibitor or inducer of the P450 system?

Ketoconazole is a strong inhibitor of P450 enzymes.

How does flucytosine work as an antifungal medication?

It is converted to 5-fluorouracil in fungal cells and works as an antimetabolite.

Why does flucytosine not kill human cells?

Human cells lack the cytosine deaminase enzyme that converts flucytosine to 5-fluorouracil.

What life-threatening toxicity is associated with flucytosine treatment?

Leukopenia and thrombocytopenia (especially in those who receive high-dose flucytosine). Non-life-threatening GI toxicity occurs more commonly.

What drugs should be used with caution along with flucytosine?

Any other medications that can cause bone marrow suppression (e.g., ganciclovir, zidovudine, anticancer medications)

How does terbinafine work?

It inhibits squalene epoxidase, another enzyme required for ergosterol synthesis.

What infections is terbinafine used for?

Dermatophyte infections. It is used topically for tinea infections and can be given orally for some onychomycosis.

How does caspofungin (an echinocandin) work?

It inhibits the enzyme D-glucan synthase and disrupts the integrity of the fungal cell wall. Since beta-D-glucans are not present in human cells, there is less toxicity and fewer drug-drug interactions.

What infections is caspofungin used for?

Fungal infection in febrile neutropenic adult patients, invasive aspergillosis, and candidemia when not responsive to other treatment

How does griseofulvin work?

Binds to polymerized microtubules and inhibits mitosis

What infections is griseofulvin used for?

Tinea

Parasitology

CHAPTER 34

Protozoa

Are protozoa single cell or multicellular organisms?	Single cell. Multicellular parasites are helminths.
What structure do protozoa typically use for motility? What is the infective life form called? What is the motile form called?	Pseudopodia (false feet) Infective form (*Entamoeba* and *Giardia*): cyst Infective form (*Cryptosporidium*): oocyst Motile form (*Entamoeba* and *Giardia*): trophozoite Motile form (*Cryptosporidium*): sporozoite
What are the four classes of medically important protozoa?	1. Sarcodina (amebas) 2. Sporozoa (sporozoans) 3. Mastigophora (flagellates) 4. Ciliata (ciliates)
Name three protozoa that infect the intestinal tract and the diseases they cause:	1. *Entamoeba histolytica* causes amebiasis. 2. *Giardia lamblia* causes giardiasis. 3. *Cryptosporidium parvum* causes cryptosporidiosis.
Name a common protozoan that infects the urogenital tract and the disease it causes:	*Trichomonas vaginalis* causes trichomoniasis.
Name some protozoa that infect blood and tissue, and the diseases they cause:	*Plasmodium* species cause malaria, *Toxoplasma gondii* causes toxoplasmosis, *Trypanosome* species cause Chagas disease and sleeping sickness, *Leishmania* species cause kala-azar and cutaneous leishmaniasis, *Babesia* species cause babesiosis, and *Naegleria fowleri* causes meningoencephalitis.

INTESTINAL PROTOZOA

How is _Entamoeba_ transmitted?	Via fecal-oral route through cysts in water
How is the intestinal lesion of _Entamoeba_ invasion classically described?	_Flask-shaped_ ulcer in the colon
How does _Entamoeba_ cause systemic disease and what is the most common organ _Entamoeba_ invades?	Invades through the intestinal wall to enter the bloodstream. _Entamoeba_ most commonly invades the liver forming abscesses.
What percentage of people infected with _Entamoeba_ become symptomatic?	Approximately 10%. Ninety percent become carriers whose feces may contain infectious cysts.
What can commonly be seen within _Entamoeba_ trophozoites?	_Entamoeba_ classically presents with engulfed RBCs in cytoplasm of trophozoites.
What patient population is at higher risk for _Entamoeba_ infection?	Men who have sex with men.
What are the symptoms of acute amebiasis?	Dysentery (bloody, mucus-containing diarrhea), lower abdominal pain, flatulence, and tenesmus
What is the treatment for amebiasis and amebic liver abscess?	Metronidazole or tinidazole. Paromomycin for carriers. Liver abscesses do not need to be drained.
What does _G. lamblia_ look like under the microscope?	The trophozoite form found in stool is pear-shaped with two nuclei and four pairs of flagella.
How is _Giardia_ transmitted?	Via fecal-oral route through cysts in water
Does _Giardia_ cause systemic disease?	No. _Giardia_ attaches to the mucosa of the duodenum, but it does not invade.
What percentage of people infected become symptomatic?	Approximately 50%. The other 50% of infected people become carriers who may continue to shed _Giardia_ cysts in their stool for years.
Among what population is _Giardia_ commonly found?	Children in day care centers, patients in mental hospitals, homosexuals engaging in oral-anal contact, and hikers drinking untreated stream water

What are the symptoms of giardiasis?	Nonbloody, foul-smelling diarrhea, nausea, anorexia, flatulence, and abdominal cramps, usually persisting for weeks to months
Besides microscopic examination of stool, how is giardiasis diagnosed?	By the string test (in which a weighted piece of string is swallowed and removed for microscopic examination for evidence of trophozoites), endoscopy (biopsy), and enzyme-linked immunosorbent assay (ELISA) (to detect antibodies) on stool specimens
How is it treated?	Metronidazole or tinidazole
How is *C. parvum* transmitted?	Via fecal-oral route through cysts in water
Does *Cryptosporidium* cause systemic disease?	No. *Cryptosporidium* attaches to the wall of the small intestine, but it does not invade.
Why is *Cryptosporidium* infection important in immunocompromised patients?	Cryptosporidiosis is usually self-limited in immunocompetent patients. In immunocompromised patients, cryptosporidiosis presents as chronic, watery, nonbloody diarrhea, and leads to large fluid losses and malnutrition.
How is cryptosporidiosis diagnosed?	Fecal smear with a modified Kinyoun acid-fast stain.
What is the treatment for cryptosporidiosis?	Supportive, nitazoxanide, spiramycin for immunocompetent patients as the disease is self-limited. No clear effective treatment is for immunocompromised patients, although there may be some benefit to start highly active antiretroviral therapy (HAART) in human immunodeficiency virus (HIV) patients.

Table 34.1 Intestinal Protozoa

Species	Mode of Transmission	Patient Presentation	Diagnosis	Treatment
Entamoeba histolytica (Amebiasis)	Fecal-oral via cysts in contaminated water	Often asymptomatic **Acute:** dysentery; lower abdominal pain; flatulence; tenesmus	Presence of cysts and/or trophozoites in fecal smear Presence of liver abscesses on abdominal CT scan or ultrasound	Metroniadazole, tinidazole
Giardia lamblia (Giardiasis)	Fecal-oral via cysts in contaminated water	Nonbloody, foul-smelling diarrhea; nausea; anorexia; flatulence; abdominal cramps	Presence of cysts and/or trophozoites in fecal smear String test Endoscopy ELISA testing for presence of *Giardia* antigens	Metroniadazole, tinidazole
Cryptosporidium parvum (Cryptosporidiosis)	Fecal-oral via cysts in contaminated water	**Immunocompetent:** self-limiting infection; diarrhea; abdominal pain **Immunocompromised:** chronic, watery, nonbloody diarrhea; fluid loss; malnutrition	Presence of oocysts in fecal smear with modified Kinyoun acid-fast stain	No treatment of immunocompetent patients

UROGENITAL PROTOZOA

How is *T. vaginalis* transmitted?	Sexual contact. There is no cyst formation in life cycle.
Where is *Trichomonas* found in humans?	Vagina. Prostate and male urethra
Approximately what percentage of women in the United States are carriers?	25% to 50%
What are the symptoms of trichomoniasis?	Watery, foul-smelling, green vaginal discharge with itching and burning. Infected men are usually asymptomatic, though some experience urethritis.
How is trichomoniasis diagnosed?	Wet mount of vaginal or prostatic fluid showing motile pear-shaped single nucleus trophozoites. Speculum may also demonstrate colpitis macularis (strawberry cervix). Vaginal pH >4.5.
How is it treated?	Treat both partners with metronidazole.

BLOOD AND TISSUE PROTOZOA

Name four plasmodia that cause malaria:	1. *Plasmodium vivax* 2. *Plasmodium ovale* 3. *Plasmodium malariae* 4. *Plasmodium falciparum*
Name the vector for plasmodia:	Female *Anopheles* mosquito
Briefly describe the life cycle of plasmodia parasite:	1. Sporozoites in mosquito saliva enter human bloodstream via mosquito bite. 2. Sporozoites enter liver cells and multiply and differentiate. 3. Merozoites are released from liver cells and enter red blood cells (RBCs). 4. Multiplication and differentiation into trophozoites and gametocytes within RBCs. 5. RBCs rupture releasing more trophozoites, merozoites, and gametocytes. 6. Mosquito picks up male and female gametocytes when ingesting human blood.

Where does sexual fertilization of plasmodia occur?	Within the gut of the female *Anopheles* mosquito
What are the various forms of plasmodia called and where are they found?	Sporozoites (found in mosquito saliva), merozoites (found in liver cells), trophozoites (found in RBCs), hypnozoites (latent form found in liver cells), and gametocytes (found in blood)
What is the classic appearance of plasmodia within RBCs?	Rings (trophozoites are ring-shaped)

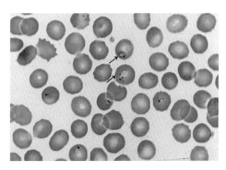

Figure 34.1 *Plasmodium falciparum* trophozoites (note the "ring form"). (*With permission from Lichtman MA, Shafer MS, Felgar RE, Wang N.* Lichtman's Atlas of Hematology. *New York, NY: McGraw-Hill; 2007. Available at www.accessmedicine.com.*)

Which plasmodia cause the most severe disease?	*P. falciparum*
What are the classic symptoms of malaria?	Recurrent fevers, chills, and sweats
Why is malaria also referred to as *blackwater fever*?	Patients may experience hemoglobinuria due to extensive hemolysis and kidney damage. The dark color of the urine gave rise to the name blackwater fever.
What are other complications of malaria?	Splenomegaly from sequestration of infected RBCs, anemia, life-threatening hemorrhage from RBC hemolysis and capillary occlusion, and cerebral malaria (hemorrhage and necrosis in the brain)
What does quartan malaria refer to?	Infection by *P. malariae*, which typically causes fevers every third day (72-hour cycle of RBC rupture). Note that many cases do not have consistent timing of fever as there is asynchronous RBC rupture.

What does malignant tertian malaria refer to?	Infection by *P. falciparum*, which typically causes fever every second day (48-hour cycle of RBC rupture). However, chills and fevers may be more erratic or even continuous.
What does benign tertian malaria refer to?	Infection by *P. vivax* or *P. ovale*, which typically causes fever every second day (48-hour cycle of RBC rupture)
Which plasmodia have a latent form?	*P. vivax* and *P. ovale*
What is the difference between relapse and recrudescence?	Relapse occurs in *P. vivax* and *P. ovale* infections and results from reactivation of hypnozoites in the liver. Of patients infected with *P. vivax*, up to 50% relapse in a few weeks to years after initial illness. Recrudescence occurs in *P. malariae* and *P. falciparum* infections and results from incomplete eradication of the parasite.
How is malaria diagnosed?	Presence of parasites in blood smear by thick and thin blood smears (gold standard in diagnosis). Thick smears examine a drop of blood and are useful for detecting the presence of parasites; thin smears examine blood smeared across the microscope slide and are useful for identifying the species of malaria.
What is the drug of choice for treating nonresistant malaria? What is the mechanism of action?	Chloroquine. Inhibits *Plasmodium* heme polymerase/hemozoin.
What drugs are available for chloroquine-resistant malaria?	Mefloquine, Malarone (atovaquone and proguanil), and quinine plus doxycycline
Why is primaquine used to treat *P. vivax* and *P. ovale* infections?	Chloroquine cannot kill hypnozoites, the latent form of *P. vivax* and *P. ovale*, but primaquine can.
What are the methods of preventing malaria?	Preventing mosquito bites (using netting or repellant), chemoprophylaxis for travelers to endemic areas

Table 34.2 Malaria

Species	Mode of Transmission	Patient Presentation	Diagnosis	Treatment
Plasmodium vivax	Insect bite (Female	Cyclical fever, chills, sweats:	Presence of parasites	Chloroquine, primaquine
Plasmodium ovale	Anopheles mosquito)	P. vivax and P. ovale— benign tertian malaria (fever every second day)	in thin and thick blood smears	Chloroquine, primaquine
Plasmodium malariae		P. malariae—quartan malaria (fever every third day)		Chloroquine **If chloroquine resistant:** mefloquine, Malarone, quinine plus doxycycline
Plasmodium falciparum (Most severe)		P. falciparum— malignant tertian malaria (fever every second day/ can be constant or mor irregular) Hemoglobinuria ("blackwater fever"— dark urine due to kidney damage) Splenomegaly, anemia		Chloroquine **If chloroquine resistant:** mefloquine, Malarone, quinine plus doxycycline

What is the definitive host of *Toxoplasma gondii*?

Domestic cats (~1% of all domestic cats in the United States are carriers) and other felines

How do humans become infected with *T. gondii*?

Ingestion of cysts in undercooked meat from animals that grazed in soil with cat feces or from contact with cat feces. Also transplacental infection of the fetus

Do asymptomatic *T. gondii*–infected individuals clear the infection?

No. The parasite tends to persist as cysts within tissues.

When do the *T. gondii* cysts typically cause symptoms?

Immunosuppression allows activation of bradyzoites within the cysts.

Will a mother infected with *T. gondii* prior to pregnancy transmit the infection to her fetus?

No. Only primary infections during pregnancy can lead to congenital infections. Infections prior to pregnancy persist in the cyst form and are not transmitted.

What are the symptoms of congenital toxoplasmosis?

Stillbirth, encephalitis, chorioretinitis leading to blindness, hepatosplenomegaly, fever, jaundice, and intracranial calcifications

How does toxoplasmosis present in immunosuppressed patients?

Typically as disseminated disease, including encephalitis

How is toxoplasmosis diagnosed?

Detection of immunoglobulin M (IgM) antibodies and multiple thin-walled *ring-enhancing lesions* (basal ganglion often affected) on computed tomography/magnetic resonance imaging (CT/MRI) (brain abscesses common in HIV patients)

Table 34.3 Trypanosoma

Species	Mode of Transmission	Patient Presentation	Diagnosis	Treatment
Trypanosoma cruzi (Chagas disease)	Insect bite (Reduviid bug/ "kissing bug")	**Acute:** unilateral painless periorbital swelling (Chagoma); flu-like symptoms (fever, lymph node swelling, malaise) **Chronic:** mega-colon, mega-esophagus, mega-cardia	Presence of trypomastigotes in blood	Nifurtimox, benznidazole.
Trypanosoma gambiese (West African sleeping sickness)	Insect bite (tsetse fly)	Indurated skin ulcer, cyclical fever spikes, lymphadenopathy, progressive demyelinating encephalitis		Suramin
Trypanosoma rhodesiense (East African sleeping sickness)				

What is the treatment of toxoplasmosis?	Sulfadiazine plus pyrimethamine
What are the three major pathogenic trypanosomes?	1. *Trypanosoma cruzi* 2. *Trypanosoma gambiense* 3. *Trypanosoma rhodesiense*
What disease does *T. cruzi* cause?	Chagas disease
What is the vector for *T. cruzi*?	The reduviid bug (kissing bug) as it bites around the mouth and eyes
What is Romaña sign?	Unilateral painless periorbital swelling ("Chagoma")
Where is *T. cruzi* found?	Central and South America, and some parts of southern United States
What tissue is most commonly infected?	Cardiac muscle
Name some other complications of Chagas disease:	Megacolon and megaesophagus from gut neuronal damage and loss of intestinal wall tone
What is the treatment of Chagas disease?	Nifurtimox or benznidazole
What disease does *T. gambiense* and *T. rhodesiense* cause and what is the vector?	Sleeping sickness. Vector is the tsetse fly.
What are the differences between *T. gambiense* and *T. rhodesiense*?	*Trypanosoma gambiense* have human reservoir and cause chronic disease. *Trypanosoma rhodesiense* have animal reservoir (commonly cattle and antelope) and cause an acute rapidly progressive disease.
How do trypanosomes continually evade host immunity?	Antigenic variation (variable surface glycoprotein)
What are the signs and symptoms of sleeping sickness? What is the treatment of sleeping sickness?	Indurated skin ulcer, cyclical fever spikes, lymphadenopathy, and progressive demyelinating encephalitis (mood changes, slurred speech, somnolence, coma). Treat with suramin and melarsoprol.

Why must treatment be initiated before the development of encephalitis?

Suramin does not cross the blood-brain barrier. However, melarsoprol is used for encephalitis.

What are the five major pathogenic leishmanias? What is the vector?

1. *Leishmania donovani*
2. *Leishmania tropica*
3. *Leishmania mexicana*
4. *Leishmania braziliensis*
5. *Leishmania major*

Vector is the sand fly.

Which *Leishmania* causes visceral leishmaniasis (kala-azar)? What are the signs and symptoms of visceral leishmaniasis?

L. donovani. Massive splenomegaly, fever, weakness, weight loss, hyperpigmentation of skin

Table 34.4 Leishmania

Species	Mode of Transmission	Patient Presentation	Diagnosis	Treatment
Leishmania donovani (Visceral/ kala-azar)	Insect bite (Sand fly)	Splenomegaly, fever, weakness, weight loss, hyperpigmentation of skin	Presence of amastigotes in skin lesion biopsy, bone marrow, spleen, liver, lymph nodes, and/or blood	Sodium stibogluconate
Leishmania tropica (Cutaneous)		Necrotic skin and cartilage uclers at bite site		
Leishmania mexicana (Cutaneous)				
Leishmania major (Cutaneous)				
Leishmania braziliensis (Mucocutaneous)		Necrotic skin and cartilage uclers at bite site Subsequent lesion formation in mucous membranes		

Which *Leishmania* causes cutaneous leishmaniasis? What are the signs and symptoms of cutaneous leishmaniasis?

L. tropica, L. mexicana, L. Braziliensis, and *L. major.* Necrotic ulcers of skin, cartilage, and mucous membranes from bite sites

What is the treatment of *Leishmania* infection?

Sodium stibogluconate

How does *Babesia* infection present?

Malaria-like symptoms because *Babesia* causes hemolytic anemia. Infections are most problematic in postsplenectomy patients.

What coinfection can occur with babesiosis?

Lyme disease because both are transmitted by the *Ixodes* tick in northeastern United States.

What is the characteristic appearance of the *Babesia* trophozoite within RBCs? What is the treatment of babesiosis?

Maltese cross
Azithromycin and atovaquone

How does *Naegleria fowleri* infection present?

Meningoencephalitis rapidly fatal (<1 week), history of swimming in freshwater, amoebas in cerebrospinal fluid (CSF)

What is the treatment for *Naegleria fowleri*?

Combination of amphotericin B, rifampin, fluconazole, miltefosine, and azithromycin.

CLINICAL VIGNETTES

A 3-year-old girl whose parents put her in day care presents with nonbloody, foul-smelling diarrhea. Her parents report she has lost her appetite and complains of stomach cramps and nausea. Upon analysis of a stool sample, you observe pear-shaped, double-nucleated trophozoites with two pairs of flagella. What are the causative organism, the disease it causes, and appropriate treatment?

Giardia lamblia causes giardiasis. Treatment is metronidazole or tinidazole.

A 26-year-old PhD student just returning to the United States from rural Brazil after 6 months of fieldwork presents with a noticeable amount of swelling around his right eye. However, upon further examination he states that the swelling around his eye is painless. He also complains of muscle aches, diarrhea, and nausea. Which protozoan is most likely responsible for these symptoms, what is the vector? What is the treatment?

Trypanosoma cruzi transmitted by the reduviid bug ("kissing bug"). Treat with either nifurtimox or benznidazole.

A 20-year-old female college student has just returned from Spring break in Cancun and presents with a watery, foul-smelling vaginal discharge with severe itching and burning. After a pelvic examination, you also observe a strawberry cervix. You diagnose her with trichomoniasis and take a vaginal swab. What organism are you looking for? What is the appropriate treatment?

Pear-shaped *T. vaginalis* trophozoites. Treat with metronidazole.

A 65-year-old woman who has the reputation as the neighborhood "cat lady" presents with flu-like symptoms. You observe ring-enhancing lesions on her CT. Name the parasite she is infected with and how you would treat her:

Toxoplasma gondii. Treat with sulfadiazine and pyrimethamine.

A 6-year-old Afghani boy presents with necrotic skin ulcers. His parents tell you that they noticed several holes in their insect nets and their son has consequently acquired several sand fly bites. What parasite is most likely involved and what is the treatment?

Leishmania tropica, L. mexicana, L. major. Sodium stibogluconate

A 34-year-old hiker who has just returned from a trip in the Appalachian Mountains presents with malaria-like symptoms. He directs you to a bull's-eye-like rash on his left thigh characteristic of Lyme disease. However, you know that the *Ixodes* tick can transmit both *Borrelia burgdorferi* and *Babesia microti*. What can you look for to determine if this patient indeed has babesiosis?

Look for the appearance of the trademark maltese cross trophozoite within RBC.

A 28-year-old man presents with bloody, mucus-containing diarrhea, lower abdominal pain, and tenesmus. You determine that he has liver abscesses and diagnose him with amebiasis. What is the appropriate course of treatment?

Treat with metronidazole or tinidazole. Abscesses do not need to be drained.

An immunocompromised female patient presents with watery, nonbloody diarrhea. A modified Kinyoun acid-fast stain reveals oocysts in her stool. What protozoan is likely responsible for her symptoms?

Cryptosporidium parvum.

A 32-year-old woman from India complains of cyclical bouts of fever, chills, and profuse sweating that seem to happen every 2 days. She also tells you that she has been diagnosed with malaria once before. What species of *Plasmodium* is she most likely infected with and how do you treat her?

P. vivax or *P. ovale*. Treat with chloroquine.

CHAPTER 35

Helminths

NEMATODES

What is another name for nematodes?	Roundworms
Name the nematodes that infect the intestinal tract and the disease they cause:	*Enterobius* causes pinworm infection; *Ascaris* causes ascariasis; *Trichuris* causes whip worm infection; *Necator* and *Ancylostoma* cause hookworm infection; *Strongyloides* causes strongyloidiasis; and *Trichinella* causes trichinosis.
Name the nematodes that infect blood and tissue and the disease they cause:	*Wuchereria* causes filariasis (elephantiasis); *Onchocerca* causes onchocerciasis (river blindness); *Loa loa* causes loiasis; and *Dracunculus* causes guinea worm infection.
Which nematodes are transmitted by ingestion of eggs?	*Enterobius, Ascaris,* or *Trichuris* **Mnemonic: EAT** eggs.
What is the most frequent helminth parasite in the United States?	*Enterobius vermicularis*
How do *E. vermicularis* infections usually present?	Intense perianal pruritus in children
What area of the gastrointestinal (GI) tract does *E. vermicularis* infect?	Large intestine.
How do you diagnose pinworm?	Diagnosis with the scotch-tape test
How do you treat pinworm?	Mebendazole, albendazole, or pyrantel pamoate
Who should be treated if a child has an infection caused by *E. vermicularis*?	The patient (child) and all family members (close household contacts)

What is the most common helminth worldwide?

Ascaris lumbricoides, the largest round worm, infects up to 25% of the world's population.

How do *A. lumbricoides* infections usually present?

Early infection presents with fever, cough, and wheezing as the larvae are migrating through the tissue. Late infection presents with obstructive GI symptoms such as cramping, small bowel obstruction, pancreatitis, and cholecystitis.

Which nematodes have a lung infiltrating phase followed by coughing and subsequent swallowing of larvae?

Ascaris lumbricoides, Necator americanus, Ancylostoma, and *Strongyloides stercoralis*

What two nematodes will not present with an elevated eosinophil count because they do not invade tissue?

1. *Trichuris trichiura*
2. *Enterobius vermicularis*

How do *T. trichiura* infections usually present?

Most cases of whipworm infection are asymptomatic and there is no pulmonary migration phase. Physical complaints may include abdominal tenderness, anemia, and rectal prolapse.

Which nematodes are transmitted by direct invasion of skin by larval forms?

Necator, Ancylostoma, or *Strongyloides*

The filariform larva of this helminth penetrates intact skin of bare feet. It can also cause a microcytic anemia and its eggs are shed in stool. Identify the helminth:

Necator americanus (hookworm)

The filariform larva of this helminth penetrates intact skin but cannot mature in humans. This infection presents with intense skin itching. What is the most likely nematode?

Ancylostoma (cutaneous larva migrans)

The filariform larva of this helminth penetrates intact skin with larvae, but not eggs, being shed in the stool. Patients may present with pneumonitis, abdominal pain, diarrhea, malabsorption, ulcers, and bloody stools; and immunocompromised patients may present with invasive disseminated infection that often coexists with gram-negative sepsis. Identify the helminth:

Strongyloides stercoralis (threadworm)

With what nematode infection will you not find eggs in stool samples?

Strongyloides stercoralis. This is the only nematode capable of replicating in the host.

What nematode is transmitted by ingestion of inadequately cooked meat containing larvae?	*Trichinella*
How do *Trichinella* infections usually present?	Patients present with fever, severe muscle pain, splinter hemorrhages, and periorbital swelling. Peripheral blood smear shows eosinophilia, and x-ray shows fine calcifications in the muscle. Serum creatine phosphokinase may also be elevated.
Which nematodes are transmitted by larvae-contaminated insect bites?	*Wuchereria, L. loa, Onchocerca,* and *Brugia malayi*
Which filarial worms can cause ele-phantiasis? How are they transmitted?	*Wuchereria bancrofti* and *Brugia.* The nematodes block lymphatic drainage. Transmitted via mosquitoes
At what time diagnosis of elephan-tiasis is made by the identification of microfilariae in blood drawn during a 24-hour period? What is the treatment for elephantiasis?	Nighttime (nocturnal periodicity). Diethylcarbamazine
What eye worm is transmitted by bit-ing flies?	*Loa loa*
What roundworm is responsible for causing river blindness and is trans-mitted by the bite of an infected blackfly?	*Onchocerca volvulus*
How do you treat *O. volvulus*?	*Ivermectin*
Name the tissue-invasive nematode that is transmitted by drinking water contaminated with larvae-infected microscopic copepods:	*Dracunculus medinesis*
How do *D. medinensis* infections usually present?	Painful skin blister/ulcer in the extremity with a visible worm inside
How is dracunculiasis treated?	Medically with niridazole. However, treatment since ancient times involves wrapping the exposed worm around a stick and slowly twisting the stick to extract the worm. This nearly eradicated disease may be the inspiration for the universal symbol of medicine, the staff of Asklepios.

Table 35.1 Intestinal Nematodes

Species	Mode of Transmission	Patient Presentation	Diagnosis	Treatment
Enterobius vermicularis (Pinworm)	Ingestion of eggs	Intense perianal pruritus	Scotch-tape test. **No** eosinophilia	Pyrantel pamoate Mebendazole Albendazole
Ascaris lumbricoides	Ingestion of eggs	**Early**: fever, cough, and wheezing **Late**: cramping, small bowel obstruction, pancreatitis, cholecystitis	Fecal smear for eggs Presence of larvae in sputum Eosinophilia	Pyrantel pamoate Mebendazole Albendazole
Trichuris trichiura (Whipworm)	Ingestion of eggs	Often asymptomatic Abdominal pain, anemia, rectal prolapse	Fecal smear for eggs. **No** eosinophilia	Mebendazole Albendazole
Necator americanus (Hookworm)	Larval skin invasion	Diarrhea, abdominal pain, microcytic anemia	Fecal smear for eggs Presence of larvae in sputum Eosinophilia	Pyrantel pamoate Mebendazole Albendazole
Ancylostoma duodenale (Hookworm)	Larval skin invasion or ingestion of larvae	Intense skin itching, diar rhea, microcytic anemia	Fecal smear for eggs Presence of larvae in sputum Eosinophilia	Pyrantel pamoate Mebendazole Albendazole
Strongyloides stercoralis (Threadworm)	Larval skin invasion	Pneumonitis, abdominal pain, diarrhea, malabsorption, ulcers, bloody stools	Presence of larvae in sputum	Albendazole Thiabendazole Ivermectin

Table 35.1 Intestinal Nematodes (*Continued*)

Species	Mode of Transmission	Patient Presentation	Diagnosis	Treatment
Trichinella spiralis	Ingestion of encysted larvae in undercooked meat (especially pork)	Fever, severe muscle pain, splinter hemorrhages, perior-bital swelling	Elevated serum creatine phosphokinase Muscle biopsy Eosinophilia	Albendazole Thiabendazole Mebendazole

Table 35.2 Blood and Tissue Nematodes

Species	Mode of Transmission	Patient Presentation	Diagnosis	Treatment
Wuchereria bancrofti and Brugia malayi	Insect bite (Mosquito)	Fever, chills, headache, painful lymph nodes; elephantiasis; tropical pulmonary eosinophilia (coughing, wheezing, fatigue)	Presence of microfilariae in blood drawn at nighttime	Diethylcarbamazine
Onchocerca volvulus	Insect bite (Blackfly)	Pruritic skin rash; river blindness	Presence of microfilariae in blood-free skin snips	Ivermectin
Loa loa	Insect bite (Deerfly or mangrove fly)	Often asymptomatic; fever, chills, painful lymph nodes; tropical pulmonary eosinophilia (coughing, wheezing, fatigue)	Presence of microfilaria in the blood	Diethylcarbamazine
Dracunculus medinensis	Ingestion of larvae-infected copepods in contaminated water	Nausea, vomiting; painful skin blister/ulcer with visible worm inside		Niridazole. Wrap the exposed worm around a stick and twist slowly to extract worm

TREMATODES

What is the another name for Platyhelminthes and name the two groups:

Flatworms
1. Trematodes
2. Cestodes

What is another name for trematodes?

Flukes

Name the medically important trematodes and the diseases they cause:

Schistosoma (blood fluke) causes schistosomiasis, *Clonorchis* (liver fluke) causes clonorchiasis, and *Paragonimus* (lung fluke) causes paragonimiasis.

The first intermediate host regarding trematode infections:

Snails

Which trematode is not hermaphroditic?

Schistosoma

How common are *Schistosoma* infections?

Quite common, estimated more than 200 million people are infected worldwide.

How does schistosomiasis usually present?

Acute schistosomiasis (Katayama fever) presents with fever, headache, malaise, and cough. Chronic cases present with hepatosplenomegaly, eosinophilia, bloody diarrhea, and granulomas/fibrosis in the liver.

What are the most common *Schistosoma* that cause human infection?

Schistosoma japonicum, Schistosoma mansoni, and *Schistosoma haematobium*

What is unique about *S. haematobium*?

Schistosoma japonicum and *S. mansoni* migrate to the mesenteric venules, but *S. haematobium* migrates to the bladder veins.

What malignancy is often associated with *S. haematobium*?

It is associated with an increased incidence of squamous cell carcinoma of the bladder and is endemic in Egypt.

What is swimmer's itch?

An intense pruritus caused by a variety of *Schistosoma* endemic to freshwater snails, typically after a swim in the Great Lakes. The itching is caused by the host inflammatory response to the dead parasites. Humans are aberrant hosts in swimmer's itch.

How does *Schistosoma* evade host defenses?

They incorporate host antigen, including major histocompatibility complexes (MHCs) and blood group antigens into their surface. They also produce factors which prevent the migration of resident skin antigen presenting cells (APCs) (Langerhan cells) from migrating to the draining lymph nodes, thus preventing the activation of the immune response.

How is schistosomiasis diagnosed?

Infection with *S. haematobium* is diagnosed by urinalysis (hematuria and/or presence of eggs in the urine). *Schistosoma japonicum* and *S. mansoni* are diagnosed by stool specimens.

What is the drug of choice for schistosomiasis?

Praziquantel

Pharmacology Correlate: What is the mechanism of action for praziquantel?

Praziquantel causes paralysis and spasm by causing a rapid influx of Ca^{2+} inside the *Schistosoma*.

Immediately following the administration of praziquantel for schistosomiasis, why is there an exacerbation of symptoms?

Death of the *Schistosoma* induces a vigorous immune response.

What is unique about *Clonorchis sinensis*?

Clonorchis sinensis infections can cause choledocholithiasis (common bile duct obstruction) and cholangiocarcinoma.

What is unique about *Paragonimus westermani*?

Paragonimus westermani infection is caused by ingesting undercooked crabs or crayfish and can mimic pulmonary tuberculosis. It causes recurrent bacterial pneumonia, and presents with fever, hemoptysis, and dyspnea.

Table 35.3 Trematodes

Species	Global Distribution	Mode of Transmission	Patient Presentation	Diagnosis	Treatment
Schistosoma					
S. mansoni (Instestine)	South America, Africa	Penetration of host skin by infectious larvae (cercariae), which eminate from their intermediate host (freshwater snails)	**Acute:** intense pruritus at site of larval penetration (swimmers itch); fever, headache, malaise, cough (Katayama fever) **Chronic:** hepatosplenomegaly, eosinophilia, bloody diarrhea/urine, granulomas/fibrosis in the liver	***S. mansoni and S. japonicum:*** Fecal smear for eggs ***S. haematobium:*** Hematuria and/or eggs in urine	Praziquantel
S. japonicum (Intestine)	Eastern Asia				
S. haematobium (Bladder)	Africa				
Clonorchis sinensis	Eastern Asia	Ingestion of undercooked/raw freshwater fish (flesh or skin) contaminated with metacercariae	Often asymptomatic. Abdominal pain, nausea, diarrhea. Choledocholithiasis and cholangiocarcinoma	Fecal smear for eggs	Praziquantel, albendazole
Paragonimus westermani	Asia, South America	Ingestion of undercooked/raw crabs or crayfish contaminated with metacercariae	Mimics pulmonary tuberculosis. Severe cough, fever, hemoptysis, dyspnea	Presence of eggs in sputum or feces	Praziquantel

CESTODES

What is another name for cestodes?	Tapeworms
Name the medically important cestodes and the disease they cause:	*Taenia solium* (pork tapeworm) causes taeniasis and cysticercosis; *Taenia saginata* (beef tapeworm) causes taeniasis; *Diphyllobothrium latum* (fish tapeworm) causes diphyllobothriasis; and *Echinococcus granulosus* (dog tapeworm) causes unilocular hydatid cyst disease
Do cestodes have GI tracts?	No, they absorb nutrients from the host's GI tract. The only helminths with GI tracts are nematodes.
How are tapeworms transmitted?	Ingestion of cysts in the flesh of the intermediate host
What are the symptoms of tapeworm infection?	Patients may complain of vague abdominal pain, nausea, weight loss, anorexia, or increased appetite
What type of host are humans when tapeworm infections are more serious?	Intermediate hosts because of cysticerci (occurs when humans ingest the eggs)
What are cysticerci? Name a few manifestations of cysticercosis:	Encysted larvae found in intermediate hosts. May manifest as blindness, seizures, focal neurologic deficits, and hydrocephalus
What is unique about *D. latum*?	Fish tapeworm can cause vitamin B_{12} deficiency and megaloblastic anemia. They average 10 m in length
What type of food is associated with *D. Latum* infection?	Raw fish
Pathology correlate: How is megaloblastic anemia diagnosed?	Increased mean corpuscular volume and hypersegmented neutrophils
Why are *Echinococcus* infections particularly dangerous?	Echinococcus cause hydatid cyst disease, which may remain as an asymptomatic cyst until it causes amass effect on an organ. Surgical excision of these cysts is also particularly challenging because cyst rupture may be associated with local spread of infection or with anaphylactic reaction to echinococcal antigens.

Table 35.4 Cestodes

Species	Mode of Transmission	Patient Presentation	Diagnosis	Treatment
Taenia solium (pork worm)	Ingestion of cysts in undercooked pork. Ingestion of eggs leads to **cysticercosis**	Often asymptomatic. Abdominal pain, nausea, weight loss, anorexia, or increased appetite. **Cysticercosis:** cysticerci in skeletal muscle, brain, and/or eyes results in blindness, seizures, focal neuroligical deficit, hydocephalus	Presence of proglottids and/or eggs in fecal smear. Eosinophilia in cases of cysticercosis	Praziquantel, albendazole, niclosamide
Taenia saginata (beef worm)	Ingestion of cysts in undercooked beef	Often asymptomatic. Abdominal pain, nausea, weight loss, anorexia, or increased appetite	Presence of proglottids and/or eggs in fecal smear	Praziquantel, niclosamide
Diphyllobothrium latum (fish worm)	Ingestion of cysts in undercooked fresh water fish	Often asymptomatic. Abdominal pain, nausea, weight loss, anorexia, or increased appetite. Vitamin B_{12} deficiency, megoblastic anemia	Presence of proglottids and/or eggs in fecal smear	Praziquantel, niclosamide
Echinococcus granulosus (dog tapeworm)	Ingestion of eggs in feces	Hydatid cyst disease. Enlargement of organs where cysts are present (liver, lungs, and/ or brain)	Presence of cysts on CT scan or tissue biopsy	Surgical excision of cysts: challenging since rupture of cyst may spread infection or induce anaphy-lactic reaction. Menbendazole, albendazole

CLINICAL VIGNETTES

A 65-year-old Egyptian ex-professional swimmer presents with hematuria, dysuria, and increased urinary frequency. After a thorough workup and biopsy, squamous cell carcinoma of the bladder is diagnosed. What is the most likely infectious cause of this cancer?

Schistosoma haematobium can cause a chronic infection that has a strong association with bladder carcinoma in Egypt and Africa. The parasite penetrates the skin and matures in bladder veins.

A 5-year-old boy has multiple night awakenings accompanied by intense perianal itching. The family physician instructs the mother to dab the perianal area with a *sticky swab* and bring it into the office for analysis. The physician finds ova with a flattened side and filled with larvae. What is the most likely helminth involved?

Enterobius vermicularis (pinworm)

A 12-year-old girl, newly emigrated from Southeast Asia, presents with abdominal cramping. She is febrile, has a dry cough, pulmonary infiltrate on chest x-ray, and a high eosinophil count in the blood and sputum. Diagnosis is made by identification of eggs in feces, and a sputum examination reveals larvae. Peripheral blood smear also shows an increased number of eosinophils. What nematode is first on your differential diagnosis?

Ascaris lumbricoides

A 37-year-old woman presents with rectal prolapse. The physician has found barrel-shaped eggs with bipolar plugs in the patient's stool. Which nematode is the most likely culprit in this case?

Trichuris trichiura (whipworm)

A 12-year-old boy from West Africa presents with an itchy *leopard* rash and worms in the eyes. What is the most likely nematode involved and what is its vector?

Onchocerca volvulus (river blindness). Vector is blackfly.

Mnemonic: river blindness from the blackfly, treat with **iver**mectin (vision is *black* when *blinded*).

A 35-year-old tourist to South America acquires a helminth infection and subsequently develops portal hypertension. What is the most likely helminth involved? Infection with which helminth can lead to pulmonary hypertension?

Schistosoma japonicum. S. mansoni can cause pulmonary hypertension. Results from fibrosis of the portal venous system and pulmonary arterioles respectively secondary to an immune reaction against the eggs of the helminth.

A 34-year-old woman who enjoys eating raw freshwater fish presents with nonspecific abdominal symptoms. Peripheral blood smear is significant for an increased mean corpuscular volume (MCV), and hypersegmented neutrophils. What is the most likely diagnosis?

Diphyllobothrium latum (fish tapeworm) with vitamin B_{12} deficiency

A 56-year-old man goes in for surgical removal of a pulmonary cyst. During the procedure, the surgeon accidentally nicks the cyst, which results in leakage of cystic fluid. Immediately after the fluid leakage, the patient goes into anaphylaxis. Which helminthic infection is responsible for these series of events?

Echinococcus (hydatid cyst disease)

A 25-year-old man presents with vague abdominal pains. The patient reveals that he eats rare pork quite often (which is inadvisable). Proglottids and eggs were found in his stool. What is the diagnosis?

Taenia solium (pork tapeworms)

A 16-year-old girl presents with nausea and vomiting. She directs your attention to a painful skin blister, and upon further examination you observe a visible worm within the ulcer. She also tells you that she has been drinking out of a local pond that may be contaminated with tiny crustaceans. What parasite is most likely responsible for her illness and how do you treat her?

Dracunculus medinensis. Treat with niridazole or manually remove worm by wrapping the exposed part around a small stick and gently twist to extract.

Immunology

CHAPTER 36

Cells and Signals of the Immune System

The two types of immunity are innate and adaptive immunity. What cells mediate innate immunity?

Monocytes/macrophages, neutrophils, natural killer (NK) cells, gamma-delta T cells

Adaptive immunity is composed of two responses. What cells mediate each response?

1. Humoral immunity is mediated by B lymphocytes.
2. Cell-mediated immunity is mediated by T lymphocytes (also macrophages, NK cells).

By which cytokine is B- and T-cell proliferation in early lymphocyte maturation stimulated?

Interleukin 7 (IL-7)

What interacts with the T-cell receptor (TCR) of an immature, double-positive T cell ($CD4^+/CD8^+$) to signal differentiation into a single-positive cell? In what organ does this occur?

Interaction with either major histocompatibility complex I (MHC I) ($CD8^+$) or MHC II ($CD4^+$) in the cortex of the thymus

What two processes eliminate immature T cells lacking proper antigen receptor specificities?

1. Positive selection selects for lymphocytes with TCRs that recognize self-MHC proteins, ensuring that only T cells with TCR that recognize MHC mature.
2. Negative selection eliminates autoreactive T cells that bind to MHC with high affinity.

What mechanism drives cell elimination in positive selection?

T cells that cannot bind to self-MHC molecules undergo apoptosis.

What process results in apoptosis of T-helper cells ($CD4^+$, Th) or cytotoxic T cells ($CD8^+$, Tc) bearing TCRs for self-proteins?

Tolerance, which prevents autoimmune reactions

What cytokine released by activated Th cells further stimulates Th-cell survival/proliferation?

IL-2. It binds to the IL-2 receptor on Th cells causing further proliferation.

Name the two signals that are needed to activate T cells:

1. The first signal is the MHC/antigen complex interaction with a TCR specific for that antigen.
2. The second is the *costimulatory* signal of the CD28 protein on the T cell with the B7 protein on the antigen-presenting cells (APCs).

What is the result of an interaction between a T cell and an APC in the absence of costimulation?

Anergy or unresponsiveness of T cells

What T-cell protein displaces CD28 from B7, inhibiting T-cell activation and ensuring T-cell homeostasis?

Cytotoxic T-lymphocyte antigen 4 (CTLA-4)

What is a consequence to T cells that lack CTLA-4?

It is thought that cells without CTLA-4 participate more often in autoimmune processes.

Which MHC class molecule presents processed antigens from organisms that have been phagocytosed? What cells possess this MHC class?

MHC-II complexes on professional APC present extracellular, phagocytosed proteins to Th cells.

What cells function as professional APCs?

Dendritic cells, macrophages, and B cells

What is the source of antigen presented by MHC-I molecules? What cells possess this class?

MHC-I complexes on all nucleated cells present intracellular proteins to Tc cells.

What is the cluster of polypeptides present in all T cells that is important in signal transduction by the TCR?

The CD3 complex

Induction of which of the T-cell helper lines (Th1 or Th2) elicits a more effective response against intracellular pathogens such as *Mycobacterium tuberculosis*?

Th1 cells are more effective against intracellular pathogens.

Which cytokine released by Th1 cells is involved in macrophage activation?

γ-Interferon (γ-INF)

What other signaling pathway results in macrophage activation?

The interaction of CD40 on macrophages with CD40L on T cells

What transcription factor is involved in both γ-interferon and CD40/CD40L signaling?	Nuclear factor-κB
How do macrophages respond to γ-interferon and CD40/CD40L signaling?	Cytokine release, increased microbicidal activity, increased phagocytic activity (through upregulation of B7 and MHC II)
Once activated, what are the major cytokines released by macrophages?	Tumor necrosis factor (TNF), IL-1 and IL-8 (leukocyte recruitment), IL-6 (lymphocyte activation), and IL-12 (Th1 differentiation)
What are the microbicidal substances produced by activated macrophages?	Reactive oxygen species, nitric oxide, and lysosomal enzymes
What are the main effector cells and cytokines of *delayed hypersensitivity*?	Macrophages induce differentiation of naïve Th cells into Th1 cells by secretion of IL-12. IL-12 acts on NK cells to produce γ-IFN which also promotes Th1 differentiation. Th1 cells in turn release γ-interferon, activating macrophages.
Against what pathogens is delayed hypersensitivity needed?	Intracellular pathogens (e.g., *M. tuberculosis*, *Salmonella typhimurium*, and *Histoplasma*)
To what families of pathogens are patients with T-cell deficiencies most susceptible?	All severe T-cell deficiencies leave patients particularly susceptible to mycobacterial, viral, and fungal infections.
How is the activation of a T cell by a *superantigen* different from that by a typical antigen?	Superantigens (staphylococcal toxic shock syndrome toxin [TSST]) bind to MHC-II protein directly and complex with the V_β chain of the TCR on Th cells. They are not processed by APCs.
What is the result of superantigen activation of Th cells?	Massive Th-cell activation and cytokine release, resulting in shock
Which cytokine induces naïve Th cells into mature Th2 cells?	IL-4
What cytokines do Th2 cells produce? What properties do these cytokines share?	IL-4, IL-5, IL-10, and IL-13. All are anti-inflammatory and antagonize Th1 cells.
Which cytokines aid B cells in antibody production?	IL-4 and IL-5. IL-4 aids in production of IgG and IgE. IL-5 aids in production of IgA.

What functions do IL-4 and IL-5 from Th2 cells serve in helminth immunity?

IL-4 induces helminth-specific immunoglobulin E (IgE) antibodies and IL-5 activates eosinophils.

Which cytokines are implicated as a mediator of asthma (airway hyperresponsiveness)?

IL-4, IL-5, IL-9, IL-13

By what two main methods do CD8$^+$ cells kill virus-infected, graft, and tumor cells?

Cytotoxic T cells can lyse infected cells or induce apoptosis.

What role in graft rejections do MHC-I molecules on allogeneic donor cells have?

They are recognized by Tc cells which can kill grafted cells.

Which mature immune cell has receptors for whole, unprocessed antigens and does not require MHC presentation?

B cells, which actually present antigens themselves via MHC II to CD4$^+$ helper cells in the process of activation, can recognize soluble or cell-associated antigens.

Which types of antigens can induce antibody production by B cells without the aid of helper T cells (i.e., *T-cell independent response*)?

Multivalent antigens (bacterial capsule polysaccharides, DNA, RNA, and lipids) bind many IgM (immunoglobulin M) molecules and cross-link IgM receptors on B cells.

Where does B-cell differentiation occur?

B cells undergo differentiation in the bone marrow.

What is the predominant antibody released in the initial stages of the primary humoral response?

IgM. Following a lag phase either IgG, IgA, or IgE appear in the secondary response.

What is *class switching* of antibodies?

The process that changes IgM to IgG, IgA, or IgE

Which antibody isotypes are considered strong opsonins?

IgM & IgG

What cells and signals are involved in class switching?

Th-cell CD40 ligand interacts with B-cell CD40, inducing the release of IL-4, IL-5, and γ-INF, which signals class switching.

X-linked hyper-IgM syndrome is an inherited disorder where the CD40 ligand on T cells is defective. How would this affect B cells?

Inability to perform isotype switching, resulting in hypersecretion of IgM

How would the same syndrome affect macrophages?

The CD40–CD40L interaction is necessary for macrophage activation by T cells. Macrophages cannot be activated, resulting in susceptibility to intracellular microbes.

What are the main steps in B-cell presentation of antigens to helper T cells?

Antigen-specific B cells bind to native antigen with membrane-bound immunoglobulin molecules. After internalization and processing of the antigen in an endosome, epitopes are presented on the B-cell surface via an MHC-II molecule where it is then presented to T cell.

One of the causes of severe combined immunodeficiency (SCID) is a lack of functional IL-7 receptors. What cells are depleted? How is immunity affected?

Since T cells require IL-7 for development, both cell-mediated and humoral responses would be diminished.

What would be different about the T cells in a patient with DiGeorge syndrome compared to that of a person without it (DiGeorge syndrome results in thymic hypoplasia)?

T cells differentiate in the thymus; abnormal thymic structure would result in a lack of T cells.

What immune cell kills infected cells lacking MHC-I proteins?

NK cells destroy infected cells that lose the ability to synthesize MHC-I proteins.

By which cytokines are NK cells activated?

IL-12 and γ-interferon

Which cytokines are responsible for the increased production of C-reactive protein during an acute-phase response in innate immunity?

IL-1, TNF-α, and IL-6 induce the liver to produce C-reactive protein.

What cytokine is chemotactic for neutrophils?

IL-8 along with a complement component (C5a)

Which cytokine has a similar function to granulocyte-macrophage colony-stimulating factor (GM-CSF)?

IL-3 is made by activated Th cells and supports the growth and differentiation of bone marrow stem cells.

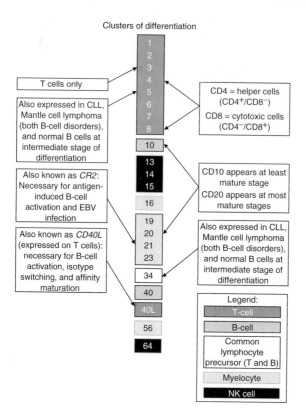

Figure 36.1   Clusters of differentiation.

Cytokine	Primary source	Primary target
IL-1	Macrophages, endothelial cells	• Endothelial cells → activation, promotes vascular permeability leading to inflammation, edema • Hypothalamus → fever • Liver → synthesis of acute-phase proteins
IL-2	T cells	• T cells → proliferation • B cells → proliferation (also may contribute to Ab synthesis) • NK cells → proliferation, activation
IL-3	T cells	• Hemopoietic stem cells → proliferation, differentiation
IL-4	Th-2 cells, mast cells	• B cells → proliferation, isotype switching to IgG, IgE
IL-5	Th-2 cells, mast cells	• B cells → proliferation, isotype switching to IgA • Eosinophils → proliferation
IL-6	APCs, Th-2 cells, endothelial cells	• Liver → acute-phase protein synthesis • B cells → increased antibody production
IL-7	Thymic stroma, marrow stroma	• Hemopoietic cells → T- and B-cell lymphopoiesis
IL-8	Macrophages, PMNs, NK cells	• PMNs → recruitment, degranulation • T cells → recruitment
IL-10	CTLs, Th-2 cells, B cells, macrophages	• Inhibits cytokine production, cellular immunity • B cells → proliferation, Ab production
IL-12	APCs	• Promotes cellular immunity • T cells → Th-1 differentiation, γ-INF synthesis • NK cells → activation, γ-INF synthesis
IL-13	Th-2 cells	• B-cells → isotype switching to IgE • Epithelial cells → mucus production • Macrophages → inhibition
IL-15	Macrophages	• NK cells → proliferation • CTLs → proliferation
IL-18	Macrophages	• NK cells → γ-INF synthesis • Th1 cells → γ-INF synthesis
α-IFN, β-INF	Macrophages, PMNs, fibroblasts	• All cells → antiviral state with increase of MHC-I expression • NK cells → activation
γ-INF	Th-1 cells, NK cells	• APCs → increase MHC-I and MHC-II expression • All cells → increased MHC-I expression and increased antigen presentation
TNF-α (cachectin)	Dendritic cells	• Dendritic cells → maturation, migration to lymph nodes • T cells → increased synthesis of IL-2 receptors • B cells → proliferation • PMNs → recruitment, activation
TNF-β (lymphotoxin)	CTLs	• PMNs → recruitment, activation

Figure 36.2   Cytokines.

CHAPTER 37

Major Histocompatibility Complex

What is the major histocompatibility complex (MHC) also known as human leukocyte antigen (HLA) complex?	Sets of highly polymorphic genes, whose final protein products regulate the immune response, especially antigen (Ag) presentation to T cells
What chromosome contains the MHC in humans?	Short arm of chromosome 6
What are the two classes of MHC? What sets of HLA genes are associated with each class? What do these individual HLA genes actually encode for?	1. Class I: HLA-A, HLA-B, HLA-C 2. Class II: HLA-DP, HLA-DQ, HLA-DR. The individual HLA genes encode for the α chain of the MHC class I molecule, and the α and β chains of the MHC class II molecule.
How are MHC inherited and expressed?	Each person has two haplotypes (two sets of MHC) with one paternal set and one maternal set expressed in a codominant gene fashion (both paternal and maternal genes are expressed).
How many MHC molecules can an individual make?	Class I: 2 MHC haplotypes $\times$ 3 HLA types = 6 Class II: 2 MHC haplotypes $\times$ 4 HLA types (DR has two β chains, either of which can pair with the α chain.) = 8

Name of the HLA haplotype(s) associated with each of the following diseases:

Multiple sclerosis	HLA-DR$_2$
Type I—insulin-dependent diabetes mellitus	HLA-DR$_3$/DR$_4$
Rheumatoid arthritis	HLA-DR$_4$
Hashimoto disease	DR$_3$/DR$_5$
Hemochromatosis	HLA-A$_3$
Graves disease	HLA-B$_8$, HLA-DR$_3$
Seronegative spondyloarthropathies (e.g., ankylosing spondylitis, Reiter's syndrome)	HLA-B$_{27}$

What is the importance of MHC classes I and II proteins?

Enable T cells to recognize foreign antigens

What is the structure of MHC class I?

Structure $= 1 \times (\alpha$ heavy chain$) + 1 \times$ (β_2-microglobin). One long chain, one short chain.

Describe the α heavy chain's structure. Where is the peptide-binding groove?

Three extracellular domains (α_1 and α_2 form the peptide-binding groove) and $\alpha_1 3$ anchors the protein to the surface of the cell by a single transmembrane domain

The β_2-microglobin is not encoded by a gene in the MHC region. What is its function?

Promotes proper folding and stabilizes MHC class I expression on the cell surface

What are MHC class I proteins and where are they found?

Membrane glycoproteins on the surface of most nucleated cells and platelets

What cells lack MHC class I proteins?

Red blood cells (RBCs), neurons, and some tumor cells

What is the function of MHC class I proteins?

They bind peptides derived from intracellular proteins (both self and foreign) and present them to cytotoxic T lymphocytes (CTLs).

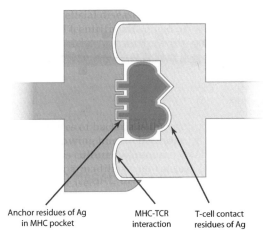

The MHC-TCR interaction is a complex interplay involving not only the identification of different portions of antigen by both receptors, but also receptor interaction with each other. The APC or somatic cell presents the antigen via MHC-II or MHC-I, respectively. The T cell's TCR then interacts with the antigen via distinct antigen residues as well as contact residues on the MHC molecule. (Note that the BCR, MHC receptor, and TCR all recognize different residues of the pathogen.)

| Anchor residues of Ag in MHC pocket | MHC-TCR interaction | T-cell contact residues of Ag |

Figure 37.1   MHC-TCR.

How do proteins become associated with MHC class I molecules?

Proteins in cytosol are routinely degraded to peptides and transported via a peptide transporter (TAP complex) into the endoplasmic reticulum, where they bind to newly synthesized HLA class I proteins.

What are sources of foreign proteins associated with MHC class I molecules? What happens to cells presenting foreign antigens?

Viruses, intracellular bacteria and parasites, or neoantigens (i.e., the cell is a tumor cell). These cells are lysed by CTLs.

What is the structure of MHC class II molecules?

Structure $= 1 \times (\alpha \text{ chain}) + 1 \times (\beta \text{ chain})$. Two equal length chains.

Describe the structure of the α and β chains. Where is the peptide-binding groove located?

Each has two extracellular domains (α_1 and β_1) and one transmembrane domain (α_2 and β_2). Peptide-binding groove is formed by the α_1 and β_1 extracellular domains of each chain.

Where are MHC class II molecules expressed?

Antigen-presenting cells—monocytes/macrophages, dendritic cells, B lymphocytes Langerhans cells, activated T cells, and activated endothelial cells

MHC class II molecules are cell surface proteins. What is their function?

Bind and present exogenous peptides to CD4+ helper T lymphocytes

How are MHC class II molecules loaded with peptide?

Vesicles containing endocytosed and cleaved extracellular protein fragments fuse with vesicles containing MHC class II molecules. In these vesicles, they are loaded onto MHC class II and are transported to the surface.

What prevents MHC class II molecules from binding peptides before fusion with vesicles containing endocytosed antigen?

The invariant chain blocks the peptide-binding groove of MHC class II molecule as it is transported through the cell. The invariant chain is degraded within the vesicle that contains processed antigen for loading.

CHAPTER 38

Innate Immunity

What are the two main functions of innate immunity?	First line of defense against microbes (e.g., skin and mucosa) and stimulates the adaptive immune response (e.g., phagocytes act as antigen-presenting cells [APCs] to induce the differentiation of T cells and secrete interleukin 12 [IL-12] to induce Th1 differentiation)
Which system is able to respond to a broader array of foreign motifs, innate or adaptive immunity? Why?	Adaptive immunity. The recombination of antigen receptor genes allows adaptive immunity to recognize 10^7 antigens. Recognition receptors used in innate immunity lack recombination ability.
Which system is better at discriminating self from nonself, innate or adaptive immunity?	Innate immunity. Adaptive immunity is responsible for autoimmunity, whereas there is no known autoimmunity associated with the innate immune system.
How does the innate immune system distinguish between foreign and self?	Innate immunity occurs in response to motifs that are characteristic of microbes but not of mammalian cells (e.g., gram-negative lipopolysaccharide [LPS], gram-positive teichoic acid, and viral double-stranded RNA).
Why have microbes not adapted to avoid the motifs recognized by innate immunity?	Innate immunity targets motifs that are indispensable to the microbe.
Name the three different epithelial layers of the human body that are considered important aspects of innate immunity:	Skin, gastrointestinal (GI) mucosa, and respiratory epithelium. Realize that the alimentary and respiratory tracts are contiguous with the external environment.

Name the three principal effector cells of the innate immune system apart from epithelial cells:

1. Monocytes/macrophages
2. Neutrophils
3. Natural killer (NK) cells

What endothelial surface structure allows *rolling* of leukocytes along the endothelial wall adjacent to infection?

E-selectins weakly bind to carbohydrate ligands on leukocytes, resulting in alternating attachment/detachment (i.e., rolling along the endothelial surface).

What endothelial surface structure allows for extravasation of leukocytes into the interstitial area of infection?

Vascular cell adhesion molecule (VCAM) and intercellular adhesion molecule (ICAM) bind strongly to integrins on leukocytes allowing for extravasation.

Mannose receptors and scavenger receptors are mechanisms utilized by which phagocyte to identify and ingest microbes?

Macrophages

How do NK cells identify infected cells?

NK cells identify virus-infected cells by failing to identify host major histocompatibility complex I (MHC-I). MHC-I molecules are normally present on the surface of host cells and inhibit NK cell killing, but are down-regulated when infected by viruses and other intracellular pathogens.

How do NK cells kill infected cells?

NK cells (and cytotoxic T cells) use perforins (create pores in the cell membrane) and granzymes (induce apoptosis).

To what types of infections do deficiencies of NK cells predispose?

Intracellular infections, including intracellular microbes and viruses

Of the three effector cells of innate immunity (macrophages, neutrophils, NK cells), which is least likely to injure host tissue?

NK cells, which only attack those cells lacking a host MHC-I. On the other hand, macrophages and neutrophils can injure host tissue via nonspecific reactive oxygen intermediates.

Which CD markers are useful for distinguishing NK cells from other immune cells? What is the function of one of these marker?

CD16 & CD56. CD16 binds the Fc region of immunoglobulin G (IgG).

Which of the complement pathways is considered part of the adaptive immune system?

The classical pathway. The alternative pathway is triggered by direct recognition of exterior features of the microbe. The lectin pathway is triggered by mannose-binding lectin, which attaches to microbial surfaces containing the mannose sugar. In contrast, the classical pathway relies on IgM, IgG1, or IgG3 to recognize and attach to the microbe and thus is dependent on adaptive immunity.

CHAPTER 39

Antibodies and Complement

What general functions do antibodies/
immunoglobulins (Igs) synthesized by
B cells perform? Define the following:

Antibodies facilitate phagocytosis by
opsonization and neutralize toxins and
viruses.

    Isotype

Antibodies that differ by constant
regions (i.e., IgG, IgA, IgM, IgE, IgD)

    Idiotype

Antibodies that differ by hypervariable
region

    Allotype

Antibodies that differ among individuals due to polymorphisms (more than
two alleles) in heavy and light chains

A simple "Y"-shaped antibody is
composed of two heavy chains and
two light chains (named according to
molecular weight) connected by disul-
fide bonds. Each chain is composed of
variable and constant regions. What are
the functions of these regions?

Variable regions of both heavy and light
chains mediate antigen binding. The
constant regions of the heavy chains
serve effector functions binding to
receptors on immune cells (e.g., IgE can
attach to mast cell receptors; IgG can
attach to natural killer [NK] cells) and
activating complement.

What are hypervariable regions?

Three sequences of amino acids with
profound variability located within the
variable regions of both heavy and light
chains. They are responsible for the
specificity of antibodies.

How many heavy-chain constant
domains (constituents of constant
regions) are present on IgG, IgA, IgM,
and IgE?

IgG and IgA have three while IgM and
IgE have four (all light chains have one
constant domain)

What are the Fab and Fc fragments? Which one is at the amino terminus and which one is at the carboxyl terminus? What separates Fab and Fc fragments?

Fab fragment is the part of an antibody that contains the antigen-binding sites located at the amino terminus. The Fc fragment, located at the carboxyl terminus, is composed of heavy-chain constant domains and serves effector functions. Fab and Fc are separated by the hinge region. In short, Fab binds antigens while Fc anchors the antibody to the cell.

What is the function of the hinge region of the immunoglobulin?

Allows flexibility within an antibody, resulting in a broader array of binding conformations

What does the identification of the presence of both κ and λ light chains suggest about a sample of antibody?

The antibodies are not monoclonal. Antibodies have either κ or λ light chains, but never both. Thus, the presence of both implies that there must be at least two different types of antibodies in the sample.

What is the function of the J chain on IgA and IgM isotypes?

The J chain plays a critical role in the stabilization of the multimeric forms of IgA and IgM. In its absence, all isotypes would be monomeric.

Define the following:

Affinity

Binding strength at a single antibody variable region and antigen epitope

Valency

Number of sites at which an antibody binds an antigen

Avidity

Overall strength of an interaction between an antibody and antigen, determined by both affinity and valency

What isotype has the highest avidity and why?

IgM, because it has 10 binding sites (i.e., valence of 10).

What isotypes of antibodies allow for B cells to achieve antigen presentation?

The membrane-bound form of IgM and IgD (which only exists as a membrane-bound form) functions to recognize and allow endocytosis of antigens within the naïve B cell, allowing them to subsequently be presented to T cells. This constitutes the recognition phase of humoral immune responses.

How does the structure of IgM in its secreted form differ from its membrane-bound form? What is the function of secreted IgM?

Membrane-bound IgM is a monomer, but secreted IgM a pentamer. IgM is the main antibody in the primary response of humoral immunity.

IgG is the main antibody in the secondary response of humoral immunity, though both IgG and IgM can opsonize. How do they differ in this regard?

IgG can directly opsonize, while IgM acts indirectly through complement activation.

Microbial pathogens entering the nasopharynx will most likely encounter which immunoglobulin isotype?

Dimeric IgA is concentrated in secretions (mucosa, tears, saliva, respiratory/intestinal/genital secretions) to neutralize microbial pathogens.

What protects IgA from being digested by intestinal enzymes?

The secretory component synthesized by epithelial cells protects IgA from proteolysis.

What two immune processes does IgE mediate?

1. Type I hypersensitivity (allergy, anaphylaxis)
2. Helminth immunity

Antibodies are found associated with the surfaces of which types of cells?

B cells (IgM and IgD, recognition phase, are membrane-bound receptors). Antibodies bind to other receptors on the following cells: mononuclear phagocytes (IgG, opsonization), NK cells (IgG, antibody-dependent cellular cytotoxicity), mast cells and basophils (IgE, anaphylaxis), and eosinophils (IgE, helminth immunity).

What isotype is most abundant in serum?

IgG

What isotype is produced in the largest amount?

IgA. About two-thirds of all antibody production is IgA, found in secretions over extensive surface area of the body.

Which immunoglobulin isotypes can initiate the classical complement cascade?

IgG and IgM both have Fc regions which are recognized by C1q—the first molecule in the complement cascade.

What is the most common immunoglobulin isotype found in fetal serum?

Maternal IgG

Why is IgG the only maternal isotype found in the fetus?

The Fc portion of the IgG molecule is recognized by a special type of Fc receptor in the placenta, thus facilitating its transfer.

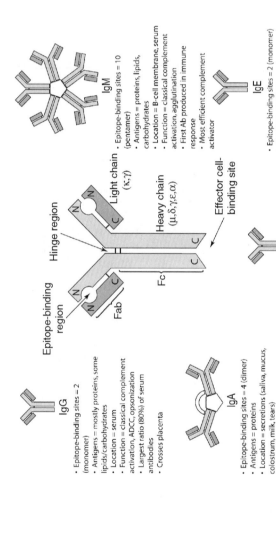

IgG
- Epitope-binding sites = 2 (monomer)
- Antigens = mostly proteins, some lipids/carbohydrates
- Location = serum
- Function = classical complement activation, ADCC, opsonization
- Largest ratio (80%) of serum antibodies
- Crosses placenta

IgA
- Epitope-binding sites = 4 (dimer)
- Antigens = proteins
- Location = secretions (saliva, mucus, colostrum, milk, tears)
- Function = neutralization/agglutination, alternative complement activation
- Most produced Ab, produced mainly in MALT
- Secretory component protects from digestive enzymes in gut/oropharynx

IgM
- Epitope-binding sites = 10 (pentamer)
- Antigens = proteins, lipids, carbohydrates
- Location = B-cell membrane, serum
- Function = classical complement activation, agglutination
- First Ab produced in immune response
- Most efficient complement activator

IgD
- Epitope-binding sites = 2 (monomer)
- Antigens = role not characterized
- Location = B-cell membrane, serum
- Function = uncertain, may control B-cell activation (self-reactive Ab)

IgE
- Epitope-binding sites = 2 (monomer)
- Antigens = proteins
- Location = mast cell/basophil membrane
- Function = opsonization, mast cell/basophil degranulation
- Immune defense against helminthes/arthropods
- Mediates allergic reactions

Light chain (κ, γ)

Heavy chain (μ, δ, γ, ε, α)

Epitope-binding region

Hinge region

Effector cell-binding site

Fab

Fc

Figure 39.1   Antibodies.

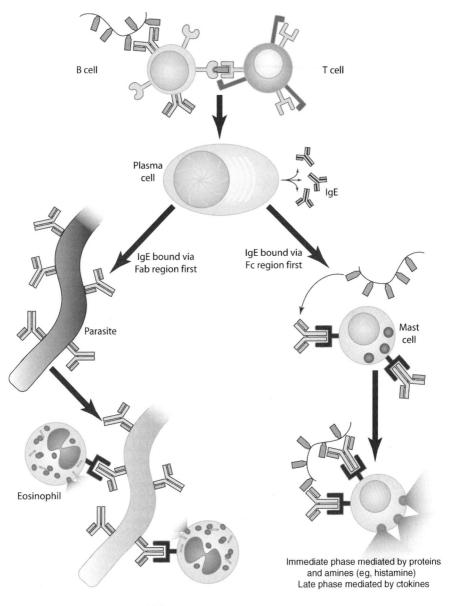

Figure 39.2   Free versus bound IgE.

Why is IgA the predominant isotype found in milk?

Again, this is due to specific Fc receptor-Fc region-mediated transfer of IgA, facilitating secretion of IgA into the breast milk.

What is the immunoglobulin isotype primarily produced by the fetus?

IgM, but the fetus also produces very small amounts of IgG and IgA

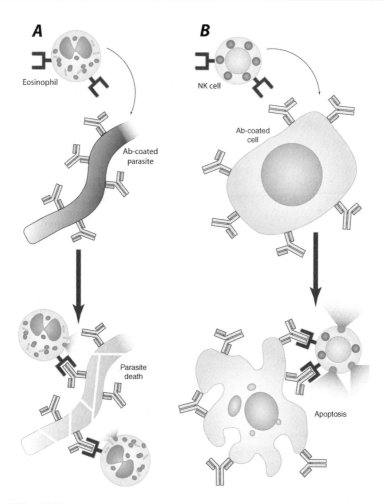

Figure 39.3   ADCC.

Define antibody-mediated cell cyto-toxicity (ADCC). What two cells utilize ADCC? What isotypes are involved in each case?

Process by which Fc receptors on a cell bind Fc portion of antigen-bound antibodies, resulting in activation of that cell.

1. NK cells via IgG lyse target cells
2. Eosinophils via IgE kill helminths

An overwhelming proportion of a single clone of IgM antibodies in serum suggestive of what disease?

Waldenström macroglobulinemia. Because IgM is the largest immunoglobulin with the most binding sites, patients with advanced disease are likely to exhibit hyperviscosity syndrome, which can lead to irreversible blindness.

An overwhelming proportion of a single clone of IgG or IgA antibodies in serum suggestive of what disease?

Multiple myeloma. Patients afflicted by this disease often exhibit punched-out lytic lesions within the bones, resulting in bone pain and hypercalcemia.

Name the three complement pathways and how they are activated:

1. The classical complement pathway is activated when C1q binds to antigen-antibody complexes consisting of IgG or IgM, or directly to the surface of certain pathogens or altered host cells.
2. The alternative pathway is activated when small amounts of C3b bind spontaneously to a microbial cell surface and then bind factor B.
3. The lectin pathway is activated by mannose-binding lectin (MBL), which recognizes mannose residues on microbial cell surfaces. MBL then triggers other proteases.

Why do free IgM or IgG not activate the complement cascade?

Binding of IgM/IgG to a microbial surface causes a conformational change to the antibody exposing the complement-binding regions.

How do IgM and IgG differ with respect to binding C1?

Only one IgM molecule is needed, whereas multiple IgG molecules are needed to bind C1q. Thus, IgM is more potent at activating complement.

C3 convertase cleaves C3 to C3a (and C3b) in each complement pathway, but how does C3 convertase differ among pathways?

Classical and lectin pathways: C3 convertase is (C4b2a).
Alternative pathway: C3 convertase is (C3bBb).

In the classical and lectin pathways what enzymes cleave C4 to C4b (and C4a) and C2 to C2a (and C2b)?

Classical: C1 (subunits C1q binds the Fc fragment, C1r and C1s are proteolytic)
Lectin: Proteases triggered by MBL.

In the alternative pathway a small amount of C3b is generated. Once C3b binds B (forming C3bB) on a microbial surface, what enzyme cleaves B?

Factor D cleaves B to Bb, converting C3bB to C3bBb (i.e., C3 convertase).

C5 convertase cleaves C5 to C5a (and C5b) in each complement pathway, but how does C5 convertase differ among pathways?

Classical and lectin: C5 convertase is C4b2a3b.
Alternative: C5 convertase is C3bBbC3b.

At which complement factor do all three complement pathways converge?

C5. Though C3 is present in all three complement cascades, it does not mark a convergence point.

What are the roles of the unbound protein fragments of the complement pathways, namely C3a, C4a, and C5a?

All three induce smooth muscle contraction and increase vascular permeability. C3a and C5a cause mast cell degranulation, leading to an anaphylaxis-like reaction. C5a also stimulates leukocyte chemotaxis and extravasation.

What is the role of the late factors of the complement cascade, C5-C9?

Responsible for generating the membrane attack complex (MAC), which forms pores into the microbe's cell membrane. These pores disrupt the osmotic gradient maintained by the membrane, resulting in swelling and rupture of the microbe.

What are the three effector mechanisms by which complement fights infection?

1. C3b and its proteolytic derivates promote phagocytosis through opsonization.
2. MAC causes the osmotic lysis of the gram-negative microbes.
3. C3a and C5a recruit leukocytes to areas of complement activation, thus secondarily stimulating various mechanisms of microbial immunity.

What is the most commonly identified human complement deficiency?

C2 deficiency

C1 inhibitor inhibits the classical pathway of complement activation, kallikrein of the kinin system, and some coagulation factors. What condition results from a deficiency of C1 inhibitor?

Hereditary angioedema is an autosomal dominant disease with edema in multiple organs, due to increased production of bradykinin. If the larynx is involved, the outcome can be fatal.

Severe pyogenic (*Staphylococcus*, *Streptococcus*) respiratory and sinus tract infections result from a deficiency in what complement factor?

C3

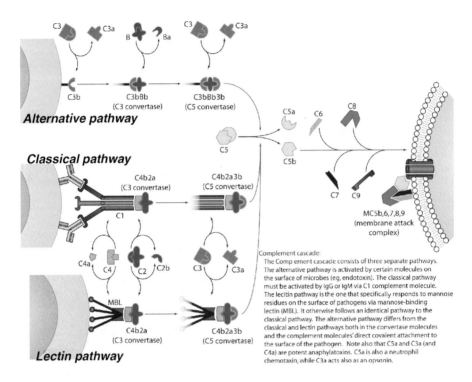

Alternative pathway

C3   C3a

B   Ba

C3   C3a

C3b   C3bBb
(C3 convertase)   C3bBb3b
(C5 convertase)

C5a   C6   C8

Classical pathway

C5

C5b

C4b2a
(C3 convertase)   C4b2a3b
(C5 convertase)

C7   C9

C1

MC5b,6,7,8,9
(membrane attack
complex)

C4a   C4   C2   C2b   C3   C3a

MBL

C4b2a
(C3 convertase)   C4b2a3b
(C5 convertase)

Lectin pathway

Complement cascade:
The Comp ement cascade consists of three separate pathways.
The alternative pathway is activated by certain molecules on
the surface of microbes (eg, endotoxin). The classical pathway
must be activated by IgG or IgM via C1 complement molecule.
The lecitin pathway is the one that specifically responds to mannose
residues on the surface of pathogens via mannose-binding
lectin (MBL). It otherwise follows an identical pathway to the
classical pathway. The alternative pathway differs from the
classical and lectin pathways both in the convertase molecules
and the complement molecules' direct covalent attachment to
the surface of the pathogen. Note also that C5a and C3a (and
C4a) are potent anaphylatoxins. C5a is also a neutrophil
chemotaxin, while C3a acts also as an opsonin.

Figure 39.4   Complement cascades.

Deficiencies in the late factors of the complement cascade, C5-C9, result in susceptibility to what specific microbes?	The *Neisseria* species of bacteria (*Neisseria meningitidis* and *Neisseria gonorrhoeae*)
What is the role of decay-accelerating factor (DAF) in the complement cascade?	DAF inhibits formation of the alternative pathway C3 convertase by competing with factor B for binding to C3b and accelerates the decay of an existing C3 convertase by displacing Bb from this enzyme.
What is responsible for the specificity of the complement cascade to microbes and not host cells?	Regulatory proteins found on host cells but not microbes inhibit complement activation. Think of microbes as lacking the *off-switch* for complement-mediated lysis.
Name two molecules that result in direct opsonization:	1. IgG 2. C3b

CHAPTER 40

Humoral Immunity

Humoral immunity and cell-mediated immunity are the two branches of adaptive immunity. What mediates humoral immunity? What are the targets of humoral immunity?

Humoral immunity is a B-cell and antibody-mediated response directed against extracellular microbial pathogens (especially encapsulated bacteria), certain intracellular microbial pathogens (viruses), and microbial toxins.

What is the difference between the recognition phase and effector phase of humoral immunity?

The recognition phase involves the identification of antigens via membrane-bound immunoglobulins (IgM and IgD) on the surface of the naïve B cell. The effector phase is characterized by secretion of immunoglobulins from plasma cells (i.e., mature B cells).

A primary response is generated when an antigen is first encountered. Second, exposure to that same antigen is known as the secondary response. What are key differences between primary and secondary responses? What accounts for these differences?

The primary response has a longer lag period (time until antibody is produced) and is typically characterized by IgM followed by low amounts of IgG. The secondary response is characterized by a faster and larger production of IgG that persists longer. These differences are due to antigen-specific memory B cells in the secondary response.

What is affinity maturation?

Process that selects for B cells producing antibodies of highest affinity to an antigen of interest through successive exposure to that antigen in the periphery

What genetic process drives affinity maturation?

Somatic hypermutation results in random and rapid point mutations in variable gene segments of V(D)J genes, modifying the affinity of a B cell's immunoglobulin. The B cells expressing immunoglobulins with highest affinities are then selected through interaction with antigen.

What is the name of the process by which immature B cells expressing immunoglobulins with a high affinity for self-antigens are restricted from becoming mature?

Negative selection. An analogous process occurs with T cells.

What type of cell stimulates B-cell clonal expansion, isotype switching, affinity maturation, and differentiation into memory B cells?

Helper T cells ($CD4^+/CD8^-$)

What are the two types of cells that may become activated B cells?

1. Plasma cells, which are responsible for secretion of antibodies
2. Memory B cells, which undergo affinity maturation and may differentiate into plasma cells upon reexposure to the antigen

Will a single antigen with a single epitope activate a B cell?

No. B-cell activation is dependent on the cross-linking of membrane-bound IgM and IgD, which requires more than one epitope. (This is true for most antigens, but there are plenty of examples of monomeric soluble protein antigens where cross-linking is not required, and T cell helps overcome this requirement.)

How do B-cell and T-cell receptors differ with respect to the native form (i.e., three-dimensional shape) of the antigen?

T-cell receptors recognize only a linear peptide sequence that results from processing within an antigen-presenting cell (APC). The B-cell receptors can recognize the native form of the antigen.

In which area of the lymphoid follicle do B-cell proliferation, early antibody secretion, and isotype switching occur?

These early-phase, T-cell–dependent responses occur in the marginal zone.

In which area of the lymphoid follicle do B-cell affinity maturation and isotype switching occur?

These late-phase events occur in the germinal centers. Isotype switching can occur in the early or late phases and in two separate locations.

What processes result from interaction of CD40 on B cells with CD40L on T cells?

Isotype switching, B-cell activation, and affinity maturation. The T-cell cytokines also play a role in these processes.

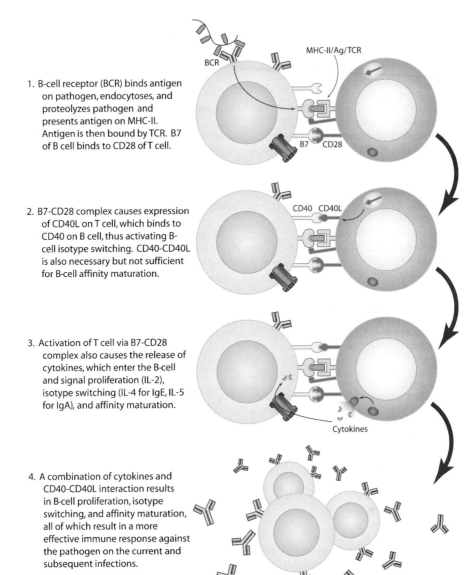

1. B-cell receptor (BCR) binds antigen on pathogen, endocytoses, and proteolyzes pathogen and presents antigen on MHC-II. Antigen is then bound by TCR. B7 of B cell binds to CD28 of T cell.

2. B7-CD28 complex causes expression of CD40L on T cell, which binds to CD40 on B cell, thus activating B-cell isotype switching. CD40-CD40L is also necessary but not sufficient for B-cell affinity maturation.

3. Activation of T cell via B7-CD28 complex also causes the release of cytokines, which enter the B-cell and signal proliferation (IL-2), isotype switching (IL-4 for IgE, IL-5 for IgA), and affinity maturation.

4. A combination of cytokines and CD40-CD40L interaction results in B-cell proliferation, isotype switching, and affinity maturation, all of which result in a more effective immune response against the pathogen on the current and subsequent infections.

Figure 40.1   B-cell activation.

The Th-2 subset of T cells, which produce IL-4, cause B-cell expression of what isotype?

IgE

TGF-β causes B-cell expression of what isotype?

IgA

What cytokine expressed by T cells also causes isotype switching to IgA?

IL-5

What is a hapten? How are antibodies generated against haptens?

Haptens are small chemicals that are nonimmunogenic by itself but can trigger an immune response when attached to a larger carrier protein. The body recognizes this new hapten-carrier protein complex as foreign and thus triggers the response. Haptens complex with a carrier protein such that T cells can recognize the hapten-carrier protein complex and activate B cells to generate antihapten antibodies.

When in conjunction with TCR-MHC II binding, interaction of the CD28 on the T cell with B7 on a B cell or other APC results in what process in T-cell–mediated immunity?

Activation of the T cell, causing the secretion of cytokines from the T cell that assist in maturation of the B cell.

CHAPTER 41

Cell-Mediated Immunity

Cell-mediated immunity (CMI) and humoral immunity are the two aspects of adaptive immunity. What mediates CMI?

T-helper cells (CD4$^+$/CD8$^-$; Th cells), cytotoxic T cells (CD8$^+$/CD4$^-$; Tc cells), macrophages, and natural killer (NK) cells

How are CMI and humoral immunity elicited by antigen? Name the major difference between them.

Unlike the IgM B-cell antigen receptor, the T-cell receptor (TCR) is not secreted. Immunity must be conferred via direct contact between cells.

Against what two major types of cells is cell-mediated immunity mainly directed?

1. Cells with intracellular microorganisms
2. Aberrant, endogenous cells such as cancer cells

To which types of infections are persons with a deficiency in cell-mediated immunity prone?

Infections with viruses, fungi, *Mycobacterium*, and other intracellular organisms

What are the two types of naïve Th cells? What are their functions?

1. Th1 cells mediate the inflammatory process and activate macrophages.
2. Th2 cells inhibit both the inflammatory process and macrophage activation and aid in helminth immunity and antibody production.

List the major steps in Th1-cell–mediated macrophage activation:

1. Antigen-presenting cells (APCs) present antigen to naïve Th cells, leading to Th1-cell differentiation and sensitization in lymph nodes.
2. Transit of Th1 cells to site of antigen release (i.e., site of infection).
3. Th1-cell activation of macrophages.

Name the different types of APCs. What two signals are needed to activate a Th cell? What cytokine do APCs secrete to induce Th1-cell differentiation?

B cells, macrophages, and dendritic cells. APC's major histocompatibility complex II (MHC-II) molecule with antigen binds to TCR/CD4 and APC's B7 protein binds to Th cell's CD28, providing the necessary costimulation for activation. IL-12 and γ-IFN differentiates naïve Th cells into Th1 cells.

Through what three signals do Th1 cells migrate to source of antigen (infection) and activate macrophages that present the antigen of interest?

1. Interaction of MHC-II with bound antigen and TCR/CD4
2. CD40 on macrophage with CD40L on Th1 cell
3. γ-IFN released from Th1 cell with γ-IFN receptor on macrophage

What are the functions of macrophages?

Macrophages present antigens, produce cytokines, and perform phagocytosis.

What functions of macrophages are enhanced in T-cell activation of macrophages?

Activated macrophages kill phagocytosed microbes via H_2O_2, $O_2^{\bullet-}$, and NO; trigger acute inflammation; and facilitate tissue repair by phagocytosis of necrotic tissue.

Delayed-type hypersensitivity (DTH, type IV) is the only cell-mediated hypersensitivity reaction. Describe it and name some examples:

Previously sensitized T cells reencounter the initial antigen and trigger macrophage activation, a process that develops over 24 to 48 hours. Examples include acute transplant rejections, tuberculosis (TB) skin tests, and contact dermatitis.

Describe the histopathology of a granuloma. In what instances are granulomas produced?

Granulomas are composed of a central core of activated macrophages surrounded by lymphocytes and are formed in response to persistent antigen stimulation of CTL (cytotoxic T lymphocytes).

Activated macrophages in a granuloma are also called epithelioid cells due to morphological changes. What cytokine triggers this change?

γ-IFN

How are Tc cells activated?

Tc cells require APC with MHC-I with antigen of interest binding to TCR/CD8 on Tc cell and costimulation by either B7/CD28 or cytokines (IL-2) from Th cells.

How do activated Tc cells recognize infected cells?

Through presentation of the antigen of interest on the infected cell by the MHC-I molecule

How do activated Tc cells kill infected cells?

Perforins (create holes in the cell membranes, disrupts osmotic balance), granzymes (activate apoptosis through caspases), and FasL on Tc cells binds Fas on target cells also resulting in apoptosis.

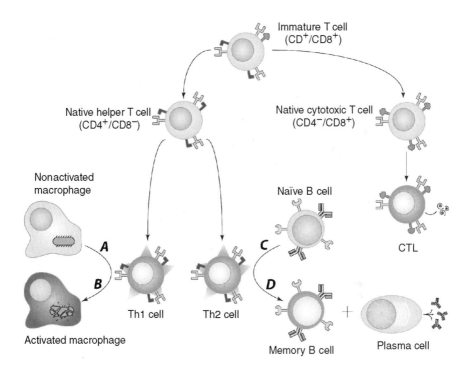

Figure 41.1   T-cell functions.

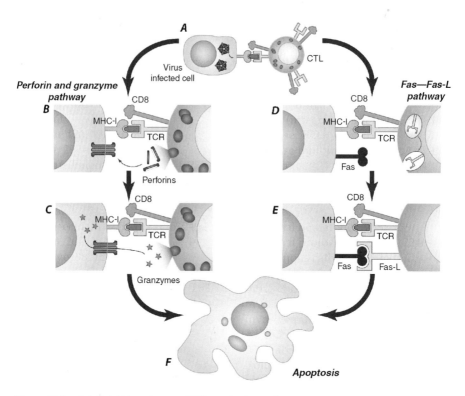

Figure 41.2   Cytotoxic T Lymphocytes (CTL) mechanisms of action.

CHAPTER 42

Hypersensitivity

Which of the hypersensitivity reactions are antibody mediated?	Types I, II, III
Which of the hypersensitivity reactions is cell mediated?	Type IV
What antibody mediates type I reactions?	Immunoglobulin E (IgE)
What antibodies mediate types II and III reactions?	IgG and IgM

TYPE I HYPERSENSITIVITY

What are type I reactions also referred to as?	Allergic reaction, immediate hypersensitivity, or anaphylactic hypersensitivity
In type I reactions, allergens (i.e., antigens) are presented to TH2 cells. The activated TH2 cells then release IL-4, IL-5, and IL-13. Describe the function of each of these cytokines in type I reactions:	IL-4: key factor that causes B cells to switch from IgM to IgE production, induces Th2-cell differentiation IL-5: activates eosinophils IL-13: promotes IgE production by B cells, induces Th2-cell differentiation of T cells, causes mucus secretion in epithelial cells, and enhances smooth muscle contraction
What are the steps of a type I reaction? Include processes that occur at the time of initial antigen exposure and the subsequent exposure.	IgE antibodies are produced upon initial exposure to allergen → IgE binds to Fc receptors on the surface of mast cells/basophils. There is no allergic reaction on initial exposure. When the individual is reexposed to the allergen the second time → the allergen causes cross-linking of bound IgE molecules → the cross-linking activates IgE-mediated degranulation in mast cells/basophils with release of various mediators the most important of which is histamine, the mediator responsible for the anaphylactic symptoms.

(1) The antigen penetrates the host's primary defenses (eg, skin, mucous), thus exposing itself to the mediators of the host's secondary defenses. This constitutes the first exposure.

(2) The antigen is recognized by one of the membrane-bound immunoglobulins on the B-cell surface. The B cell internalizes, processes, and expresses a portion of the antigen via MHC-II receptors. Presentation of the antigen by the MHC-II to the TCR of the T cell results in activation of Th-2 cells, which produce several cytokines, including IL-2 (T- and B-cell proliferation) and IL-4 (B-cell affinity maturation and production of IgE).

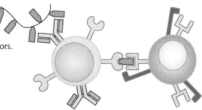

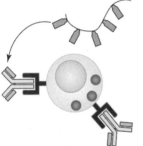

(3) The B cells then become immunoglobulins secreting machines known as plasma cells, pumping out vast quantities of a single immunoglobulins isotype. In the case of hypersensitivity, the IgE isotype is of particular interest.

(4) Mast cells contain many vesicles filled with the mediators of hypersensitivity reactions intracellularly. Extracellularly, these cells express FcεR1 receptors, which bind to the Fc portions of IgE prior to second antigen exposure. At this point, the mast cell may be considered "charged" with the potential to instigate a hypersensitivity reaction.

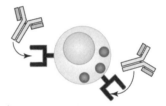

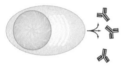

(5) Upon second exposure to the antigen, the IgE molecules bound to the charged mast cell, recognize and bind the same portions of the antigen.

(6) Antigen-bound IgE molecules cause cross-linking of mast-cell FcεR1 molecules, resulting in "activation" and subsequent degranulation of mast cells. The granules released into the interstitium constitute the fuel for hypersensitivity reactions and can be generalized into two types.
　　Immediate-phase hypersensitivity is mediated by proteins and amines (eg, histamine) and results in the classic "wheal and flare" reaction in minutes after exposure.
　　Late-phase hypersensitivity is mediated by cytokines, which induce a storm of inflammatory leukocytes (eg, neutrophils, eosinophils, basophils) 2-4 hours after the immediate phase. Inflammation typically peaks at 24 hours and subsides gradually thereafter.

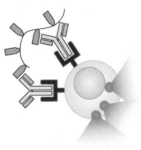

Figure 42.1　Hypersensitivity.

Type I reactions involve both primary and secondary mediators. Explain the difference between the two.	Primary mediators: preformed molecules stored in granules that are directly released Secondary mediators: generated de novo as a consequence of mast cell/basophil activation

Histamine and proteases/hydrolases are primary mediators. What are their functions?

Histamine: vasodilation, increases vascular permeability and plasma leak (edema formation), smooth muscle contraction increases secretions (nasal, respiratory)
Proteases/hydrolases: tissue damage, activate complement, cleavage of membrane receptors

Leukotrienes B4, C4, D4, and E4, and cytokines are secondary mediators. What are their functions?

Leukotrienes: B4 → recruits white blood cell (WBC). C4/D4/E4 → vasodilation, increases vascular permeability
Cytokines: mediate the inflammatory response of the late phase (see below)

What are the two phases of type I hypersensitivity reactions?

1. Immediate phase: rapid degranulation of preformed mediators in mast cells/basophils within minutes of reexposure to antigen that cross-links the cell-bound IgE
2. Late phase: 2 to 48 hours after antigen exposure; secondary mediators cause an influx, maturation, and activation of inflammatory cells and increase their survival in tissue

What are the symptoms of the immediate phase of type I reactions?

Edema, erythema, *wheal and flare* reaction in the skin, itching (skin, eye, nose), runny nose, wheezing

What are the symptoms of the late phase of type I reactions?

Edema and induration (firmness due to increased tissue density), wheezing

What are the common clinical manifestations of type I hypersensitivity reactions?

Skin: urticaria (hives), eczema
Airways: rhinitis, asthma
Eyes: conjunctivitis

What are the consequences of IgE-mediated responses in the gastrointestinal (GI) tract, airways, and blood vessels?

GI tract: increased fluid secretion, increased peristalsis → expulsion of GI tract contents (diarrhea, vomiting)
Airways: decreased diameter, increased mucus secretion → expulsion of contents (phlegm, coughing)
Blood vessels: increased blood flow, increased permeability → edema, inflammation, and increased lymph flow takes antigen to lymph nodes

What is the most severe form of type I hypersensitivity reactions?

Systemic anaphylaxis, which manifests as life-threatening bronchoconstriction and systemic vasodilation (e.g., hypotensive shock)

What are some common causes of anaphylaxis?

Peanut, bee venom, drug, and latex allergy

What drugs are commonly given to prevent anaphylactic reactions?

Antihistamines, corticosteroids, and cromolyn sodium. Epinephrine can be given as treatment for anaphylactic reactions.

How does cromolyn sodium work on mast cells?

It stabilizes mast cell membranes preventing degranulation.

What do patients with atopic disorders (asthma, eczema, and urticaria) have elevated levels of?

IgE, Th2 cytokines

Drugs commonly cause hypersensitivity reactions by acting as haptens. What is a hapten and how does this induce hypersensitivity reactions?

A hapten is a molecule, which, by itself, cannot induce an immune response. The hapten, usually a drug or its metabolite, binds to an endogenous protein that then induces antibody formation. The antibody reacts to the hapten (drug or its metabolite) upon subsequent exposure.

TYPE II HYPERSENSITIVITY

What are type II hypersensitivity reactions also known as?

Cytotoxic hypersensitivity

What reaction occurs in type II hypersensitivity?

Antibodies against endogenous cell membrane antigens fix complement causing complement-mediated lysis via membrane attack complex.

For each disease associated with type II hypersensitivity, name the target:

Warm/cold autoimmune hemolytic anemia	Self-RBC membrane proteins (warm = IgG; cold = IgM)
Erythroblastosis fetalis	Fetal D-Rh antigen
Pernicious anemia	Intrinsic factor (binds B12)
Antineutrophil cytoplasmic antibodies (ANCA) vasculitis	Neutrophil granule proteins
C-ANCA	PR3
P-ANCA	Myeloperoxidase
Goodpasture syndrome	Alveolar and glomerular basement membranes
Rheumatic fever	Myocardial antigens that cross-react with streptococcal antigens (possibly the *Streptococcus* M protein)
Graves disease	Thyroid-stimulating hormone (TSH) receptor
Myasthenia gravis	Acetylcholine receptor
Lambert-Eaton myasthenic syndrome	Presynaptic Ca^{2+} channels
Pemphigus vulgaris	Epidermal desmosomes
Bullous pemphigoid	Epidermal-dermal hemi-desmosomes

What drugs are associated with warm autoimmune hemolytic anemia? Of these, which drug(s) are associated with haptens? Which drug(s) generate autoantibodies?

Penicillin and quinidine are hapten forming. α-Methyl dopa generates autoantibodies.

What test is positive in warm autoantibody disease?

Direct antiglobulin (Coombs) test

Cold autoimmune hemolytic disease has an acute and chronic form. What infections are associated with the acute form? What type of neoplasm is associated with the chronic form?

Acute form is associated with *Mycoplasma pneumoniae* and infectious mononucleosis (e.g., Epstein-Barr virus [EBV]). Chronic form is associated with lymphoid neoplasms.

How is the autoantibody in Graves disease different from other autoantibodies?

The autoantibody in Graves disease, a thyroid-stimulating immunoglobulin (TSI), actually binds and activates the TSH receptor.

What type II disease is mediated by an autoantibody that shares the same target as exfoliatin (*Staphylococcus* toxin in scaled skin syndrome)?

Pemphigus vulgaris

What region of the autoantibodies attaches to the antigen in type II reactions? What region binds the complement?

IgG or IgM attaches to the antigen at their Fab region and attaches complement at their Fc region.

TYPE III HYPERSENSITIVITY

What are type III hypersensitivity reactions also known as?

Immune complex hypersensitivity

In type III reaction, formation of large antigen-antibody immune complexes deposit into tissues and fix complement. How does activation of complement result in tissue damage? How does this differ from type II hypersensitivity?

Complement activation recruits neutrophils, which release proteolytic enzymes and cause tissue damage. This differs from type II hypersensitivity in which tissue damage is caused by autoantibody-mediated complement activation (not by formation of large immune complexes).

One important factor that determines if antigen-antibody complexes deposit into tissue is the relative amount of antigen versus antibody. Why do antigen-predominant complexes typically form pathogenic deposits?

Antigen-antibody complexes are cleared when mononuclear phagocytes bind to antibody, resulting in endocytosis of the complex. In antigen-predominant complexes, fewer antibodies means less clearance and a propensity to form pathogenic deposits.

What is a pathology term used to describe type III inflammation in vessels?

Fibrinoid necrosis (eosinophilic staining accumulation)

What are the two typical type III hypersensitivity reactions?

1. Arthus reaction: local deposition of immune complexes.
2. Serum sickness: systemic inflammatory response to immune complexes deposits throughout the body.

Describe how an Arthus reaction is evoked:

Antigen is subcutaneously injected into a host with preformed antibodies to this antigen causing local edema and possible ulceration. Often presented on exams as a reaction secondary to vaccines. Considered a type III hypersensitivity reaction due to immune complex formation and deposition.

Hypersensitivity pneumonitis (*farmer lung*) is an Arthus reaction caused by inhalation of what bacteria?

Thermophilic actinomycetes

What is the typical clinical presentation of serum sickness?

Fever, hives, arthralgia, lymphadenopathy, splenomegaly, and eosinophilia appear days to weeks after antigen exposure.
Mnemonic: Serum Sickness **HEALS** For Weeks (**H**ives, **E**osinophilia, **A**rthralgia, **L**ymphadenopathy, **S**plenomegaly, **F**ever).

What drug is associated with serum sickness?

Penicillin. Note that penicillin can cause types I, II, and III via hapten formation.

What are well-known diseases that are resulted from type III immune-complex deposition?

Poststreptococcal glomerulonephritis, rheumatoid arthritis, and systemic lupus erythematosus

TYPE IV HYPERSENSITIVITY

What are type IV hypersensitivity reactions also known as?

Delayed-type hypersensitivity (DTH)

What are the two types of type IV hypersensitivity?

1. Classic (tuberculin-like) DTH
2. Contact dermatitis

In the first step of classic DTH, macrophages present antigens to CD4$^+$ helper cells and induce CD4$^+$ cells to become what specific subtype? What cytokine secreted by macrophages drives this process?

Macrophages induce CD4$^+$ T cells to mature into Th1 cells. IL-12 is the cytokine that drives this process.

These Th1 cells often remain in the circulatory system as memory cells. When the body is exposed to the antigen for a subsequent time, what cells do these Th1 cells activate? What cytokine secreted by the Th1 cells drives this process?

Th1 cells activate macrophages. γ-IFN is the cytokine that drives this process.

What functions are enhanced when a macrophage is activated?	Increased phagocytosis, increased antimicrobial potency, increased antigen presentation, and further induction of inflammation
What is seen histopathologically in classic DTH?	Granuloma: central core of epithelioid cells (type of γ-IFN activated macrophages) with a rim of lymphocytes
Which pathogens trigger classic DTH?	Mycobacteria and fungi
A positive tuberculin skin test is a classic DTH. Describe how a positive test presents:	Minimal change in the first few hours followed by erythema and in duration of 48 to 72 hours
What are common contact allergens?	Plants (poison ivy/oak), chemicals, soaps, jewelry metal, topical drugs
What are the common symptoms of contact dermatitis?	Erythema, pruritus, and necrosis of skin with formation of large blisters within 24 hours

TRANSPLANT IMMUNITY

What is the role of MHC class II proteins on donor cells in graft rejection?	Recognized by helper T cells of the host → proliferation, cytokine production, and "help" to activate cytotoxic T cells to kill the donor cells
What are the immunological contraindications to organ transplantation?	ABO blood group incompatibility, presence of preformed human leukocyte antigen (HLA) antibodies in the recipient's serum
What does a lymphocyte cross-match do?	Screens for recipient anti-HLA antibodies against donor lymphocytes
What are the typical mechanisms by which transplant recipients are presensitized to donor antigens?	Pregnancy, previous transplantation, blood transfusion

What are the four different classes of grafts?	1. Allograft (same species) 2. Isograft or syngeneic graft (monozygotic twins) 3. Autograft (same individual) 4. Xenograft (transplant between species)
What are the three rejection reactions?	1. Hyperacute rejection 2. Acute rejection 3. Chronic rejection
What is the time frame of hyperacute rejection?	Minutes to hours
What mediates hyperacute rejection and what is the specific target on the graft?	Preformed antibodies against graft vascular endothelial antigens
What are the cellular results of hyperacute rejection?	Complement activation leading to endothelial damage, neutrophilic inflammation, and thrombosis
How can hyperacute rejection be avoided?	Matching and cross-matching the ABO blood group of donor and recipient
What is the time frame of acute rejection? What if the recipient is treated with immunosuppressive therapy?	Within days of transplantation in a nonimmunosuppressed recipient. If immunosuppressed, rejection may occur after months to years.
What mediates acute rejection and what are the targets of this response?	1. T-cell–mediated response ($CD4^+$ and $CD8^+$) to donor vasculature and parenchyma 2. Humoral rejection with antibodies against vasculature
How does each T cell participate in acute rejection?	$CD8^+$ cytotoxic T lymphocyte (CTL) recognizes and directly kills donor cells. $CD4^+$ Th1 cells mediate a DTH (type IV) response.

What causes the delay in acute rejection versus hyperacute rejection?

Time lag is due to T-cell activation/differentiation and antibody production.

Accelerated acute rejection occurs when a second allograft from the same donor is given to a sensitized recipient. What is the principal mediator of this process?

The presence of memory (presensitized) T cells

How long does accelerated acute rejection take?

5 to 6 days in the absence of immunosuppression

What is the time frame for chronic rejection?

Months to years

What is the main pathologic finding of chronic rejection?

Atherosclerosis of vascular endothelium and proliferation of intimal smooth muscle cells

What cell causes the vascular pathology that develops in chronic rejection?

It is unclear, but is a mixture of immune- and nonimmune-mediated processes.

What is the hypothesized cause of chronic rejection?

Damage of the allograft during transplant, drug toxicity, and incompatibility of minor histocompatibility antigens

What causes minor histocompatibility mismatches between the donor and recipient?

Polymorphic self-antigens: self-proteins that differ in amino acid sequence between individuals

What are the drugs used for postoperative immunosuppression?

Calcineurin inhibitors: cyclosporine and tacrolimus
Cell cycle inhibitors: azathioprine and mycophenolate mofetil
Glucocorticoids: prednisone
Antilymphocyte antibodies: OKT3, Thymoglobulin mTOR inhibitors: rapamycin

What is the mechanism behind the use of OKT3?

Antibody directed against CD3 which is found on all T cells, leading to decreased T-cell numbers

How are cyclosporine and tacrolimus immunosuppressive?

Cyclosporine prevents the activation of T cells by inhibiting the calcineurin phosphatase which blocks the synthesis of IL-2 and IL-2 receptor.

How is azathioprine immunosuppressive?

Azathioprine is an inhibitor of purine synthesis, thus blocking DNA replication and the proliferation of T cells.

What are some of the problems associated with immunosuppressive therapy?

Drug toxicities, kidney damage, increased viral infections (e.g., cytomegalovirus [CMV], herpes simplex virus [HSV]), increased viral-associated malignancies (e.g., EBV), and other opportunistic infections

What complication is of particular concern in bone marrow transplants?

Graft versus host disease (GVHD) reaction: T cells in the transplanted marrow react against alloantigens of the immunocompromised host.

What are the three requirements for GVHD to occur?

1. The graft must contain immunocompetent T cells.
2. The host must be immunocompromised so that the graft T cells are not destroyed.
3. The recipient must express antigens foreign to the donor.

How can GVHD occur even when the donor and recipient have identical classes I and II MHC proteins?

Differences in minor histocompatibility antigens

What treatments reduce the likelihood of GVHD?

Treating the donor tissue with antithymocyte globulin or monoclonal antibodies before grafting and using cyclosporine or other drug prophylaxis against GVHD after transplant

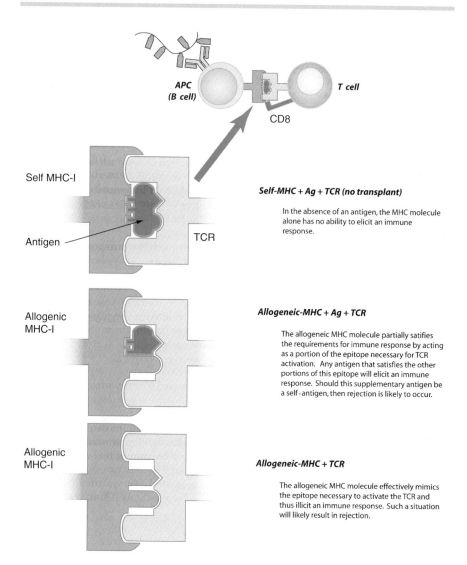

Self-MHC + Ag + TCR (no transplant)

In the absence of an antigen, the MHC molecule alone has no ability to elicit an immune response.

Allogeneic-MHC + Ag + TCR

The allogeneic MHC molecule partially satifies the requirements for immune response by acting as a portion of the epitope necessary for TCR activation. Any antigen that satisfies the other portions of this epitope will elicit an immune response. Should this supplementary antigen be a self-antigen, then rejection is likely to occur.

Allogeneic-MHC + TCR

The allogeneic MHC molecule effectively mimics the epitope necessary to activate the TCR and thus illicit an immune response. Such a situation will likely result in rejection.

Figure 42.2   Transplant rejection.

CHAPTER 43

Tolerance and Autoimmunity

Define tolerance. Why is tolerance medically important?

Tolerance is the unresponsiveness of the immune system to antigen developed upon previous exposure to that antigen. Self-tolerance is tolerance to self-antigens and autoimmune diseases occur when self-tolerance fails.

Where do the most self-tolerance-sensitive stages of lymphocyte maturation occur and why? What form of tolerance is this known as?

Central lymphoid organs, the thymus (T cells) and bone marrow (B cells), have high concentrations of self-antigens to present to immature lymphocytes. This is known as central tolerance.

What are the two central lymphoid organs?

Thymus and bone marrow.

What is the principal mechanism of central tolerance?

Apoptotic cell death (clonal deletion) of self-reactive lymphocytes

In central tolerance, immature lymphocytes with high-affinity receptors for self-antigens are deleted. What is this process called?

Negative selection

The autoimmune regulator (AIRE) gene encodes a protein that stimulates expression of endocrine self-antigens in thymic epithelial cells. If there is a mutation in the AIRE gene, what disease results?

Failure of negative selection leads to immune-mediated injury to multiple endocrine organs (autoimmune polyendocrine syndrome)

Where does peripheral tolerance occur?

Peripheral tolerance occurs outside the thymus/bone marrow.

What mechanism(s) mediate peripheral tolerance?

Peripheral tolerance is primarily mediated by the concept of anergy: T and B cells' requirement of a costimulatory signal when presented with an antigen. Without the costimulatory signals, the cells cannot be activated. Another mechanism is the production of regulatory T-cells.

What are the two requirements for CD4$^+$ helper T-cell activation?

1. T-cell receptor (TCR) must bind to major histocompatibility complex class II (MHC-II) with the antigen peptide.
2. T cell CD28 must bind to antigen-presenting cell (APC) B7 molecule for costimulation.

What happens when peptide antigens are presented to CD4$^+$ T cells by APCs deficient in costimulators? Why is this important to self-tolerance?

Anergy or unresponsiveness. Clonal anergy refers to unresponsiveness of self-reactive T cells and is an important mechanism of peripheral self-tolerance.

Anergic T cells are defined as those that fail to produce which growth factor?

Interleukin 2 (IL-2)

What differentiates clonal ignorance from clonal anergy?

In clonal ignorance, self-reactive T cells ignore self-antigens but are still functional. Clonal anergy results in permanent antigen nonresponsiveness.

Which T-cell coreceptor delivers inhibitory signals when it interacts with B7?

Cytotoxic T-lymphocyte antigen 4 (CTLA-4) (either lack of costimulation or interaction of CTLA-4-B7 at the same time as antigen results in T-cell anergy)

Repeated stimulation of CD4$^+$ T cells by antigen results in the coexpression of which receptor and ligand for activation-induced cell death?

Fas/FasL (which activate the caspase cascade via caspase 8)

What lineage of cell may also induce T-cell tolerance?

Regulatory T cells (exact type unknown) are also thought to play a role in tolerance.

Central B-cell tolerance is most likely to occur with a central antigen of what structure? Name two examples of these self-antigens:

Multivalent antigens that can bind and cross-link many receptors on each specific B cell.
1. Membrane molecules, DNA
2. Polysaccharides

What is the process by which immature B cells that encounter self-antigen in bone marrow acquire new antigen specificity for their B-cell receptors?

Receptor editing allows B cells to ignore self-antigens.

What is the fate of mature B cells that recognize self-antigen in peripheral tissue in the absence of specific helper T cells?

Anergy with exclusion from lymphoid follicles

What happens when IgG produced by B cells forms complexes with antigen and binds to their own Fc receptors?	Inhibitory feedback
What are the major factors that contribute to the development of autoimmunity?	Genetic susceptibility, environmental factors (mainly bacteria, viruses), hormonal factors (majority occur in women)
Which family of genes is most strongly associated with autoimmunity?	Human leukocyte antigen (HLA) genes
What is epitope spreading?	When autoimmune reactions against a self-antigen cause release of other self-antigens from damaged tissue, resulting in an immune response to those antigens and exacerbation of disease
Define molecular mimicry:	Antigens of a microbe induce production of antibodies that cross-react with self-antigens.
How might inflammation, ischemic injury, or trauma lead to autoimmunity?	Exposure of self-antigens that are normally concealed from immune system
What are the examples of anatomically sequestered antigens?	Intraocular proteins, sperm proteins, central nervous system (CNS) proteins such as myelin
Which autoimmune diseases are due to antibodies against receptors?	Myasthenia gravis, Graves disease, Lambert-Eaton myasthenic syndrome
What is an example of a T-cell–mediated autoimmune disease?	Multiple sclerosis, Type I diabetes mellitus, celiac disease (even though autoantibodies are found)
Which organisms are associated with reactive arthritis (previous known as Reiter syndrome?	*Chlamydia*, *Shigella*, and other enteric pathogens
Which syndrome is associated with diarrhea caused by *Campylobacter jejuni* and antibodies against myelin protein?	Guillain-Barré, also known as acute inflammatory demyelinating polyneuropathy
Which disease is associated with IgM autoantibodies formed against IgG?	Rheumatoid arthritis. Rheumatoid factors are IgM autoantibodies against the Fc fragment of IgG antibodies.
Which antibody is most specific for rheumatoid factor?	Anti-cyclic citrullinated peptide antibodies. (Anti-CCP)

What antibodies are found in systemic lupus erythematosus (SLE)?

Antinuclear antibody (highly sensitive), Anti-double-stranded DNA (highly specific), anti-Smith (nuclear ribonucleoproteins) (highly specific)

What drugs are associated with drug-induced lupus? What is the autoantibody involved in pathogenesis?

Hydralazine, procainamide, quinidine, isoniazid. Antihistone antibody **Mnemonic:** **Q**uietly **I**nduce **H**armful **P**athology (**Q**uinidine, **I**soniazid, **H**ydralazine, **P**rocainamide)

What disease is classically associated with anti-SS-B (La) and anti-SS-A (Ro) antibodies? What are the clinical symptoms?

Sjögren syndrome. It has a classic triad of dry eyes (xerophthalmia), dry mouth (xerostomia), and rheumatoid arthritis.

What disease with a complication of heart block is also associated with anti-SS-B (La) and anti-SS-A (Ro) antibodies?

Neonatal Lupus

Scleroderma results in marked fibrosis of tissue. What are the two forms of scleroderma and what are the autoantibodies associated with each one?

1. Diffuse: involves the skin and visceral organs such as the lungs (pulmonary fibrosis) and kidney vasculature (kidney failure and death). Anti-Scl-70 antibodies
2. Limited (**CREST** syndrome): **C**alcinosis, **R**aynaud phenomenon, **E**sophageal dysmotility, **S**clerodactyly, and **T**elangiectasia. Anticentromere antibodies

Which autoimmune disorder targets hair follicles?

Alopecia areata leads to variable hair loss.

Goodpasture syndrome, unlike most autoimmune disorders, is more prevalent in men. Name the autoantibody targets and resulting symptoms:

Targets the glomerular and alveolar basement membranes leading to hemoptysis and hematuria

In Goodpasture syndrome, what immunofluorescence pattern is seen on the glomerular basement membrane?

Linear pattern

Myositis, such as polymyositis and dermatomyositis, may be associated with what antibody?	Anti-Jo1 antibody (Jo1 is tRNA synthase) is often seen in polymyositis with interstitial lung disease.
Autoimmune hepatitis is a rare autoimmune disease. What antibody is detected?	Antismooth muscle antibody
What antibody is associated with primary biliary cholangitis?	Anti-mitochondrial antibody

For each HLA allele, list associated autoimmune diseases:

DR2	Multiple sclerosis, Goodpasture syndrome, SLE
DR3	SLE, diabetes mellitus type 1, celiac sprue
DR4	Diabetes mellitus type 2, pemphigus vulgaris, rheumatoid arthritis

What are the HLA-B27-associated disorders?	Ankylosing spondylitis, reactive arthritis (Reiter syndrome), inflammatory bowel disease, psoriatic arthritis **Mnemonic:** HLA-B27 **I**ncludes **R**eal **A**utoimmune **P**roblems (**I**nflammatory bowel disease, **R**eactive arthritis (Reiter syndrome), **A**nkylosing spondylitis, **P**soriatic arthritis)
Name two autoimmune diseases and one bacterial infection associated with an increased risk for B-cell mucosa-associated lymphoid tissue (MALT) lymphoma:	Sjögren syndrome, Hashimoto thyroiditis, and *Helicobacter pylori* infection
What autoimmune disease is linked with enteropathy-associated T-cell lymphoma?	Celiac sprue

CHAPTER 44

Immunodeficiency

What immune cell deficiency presents with recurrent infections with encapsulated bacteria such as *Staphylococcus* and *Haemophilus influenzae*?	B-cell deficiency
What immune cell deficiency presents with recurrent fungal, viral, or protozoal infections?	T-cell deficiency
X-linked hypogammaglobulinemia (Bruton agammaglobulinemia) has low levels of all immunoglobulins due to what underlying deficiency?	Deficiency of B-cell tyrosine kinase receptors, leading to failure of differentiation of pre-B cells into mature B cells
How does Bruton agammaglobulinemia manifest clinically?	Recurrent bacterial infections
Who typically gets Bruton agammaglobulinemia and why?	Young boys due to the X-linked recessive inheritance
How is Bruton agammaglobulinemia treated?	Treat with pooled immunoglobulin (Ig). **Mnemonic:** Bruton **He X-iBITS** (exhibits) Immunodeficiency (**He** = Boys, **X**-linked, **B**acterial infections, **I**mmunoglobulins are low, **T**yrosine kinase gene, **S**ix months = start of symptoms)
At what age do most congenital B-cell immunodeficiencies manifest?	About 6 months, as levels of maternal IgG acquired transplacentally during the fetal period begin to fall

What is the most common selective immunoglobulin deficiency, and how do patients present?

Selective IgA deficiency causes recurrent sinus and lung infections (recall IgA is typically present in mucous).

What can occur when patients with selective IgA deficiency receive a blood transfusion?

Anaphylactic reaction if the patients have anti-IgA antibodies that react against IgA in the donor serum

What embryologic process is defective in DiGeorge syndrome?

Development of third and fourth pharyngeal arches, and subsequent aplasia of thymus (third arch) and parathyroids (third arch: inferior parathyroids, fourth arch: superior parathyroid)

What immune deficiency is part of DiGeorge syndrome and how is it treated?

Deficit of T cells due to thymic aplasia results in fungal, viral, and protozoal infections (e.g., *Pneumocystis* pneumonia [PCP] and *Candida albicans*). Treat with fetal thymic transplant.

What electrolyte disturbance is seen in DiGeorge syndrome?

Hypocalcemia (and tetany) due to failure of parathyroid development **Mnemonic:** CATCH-22: Cardiac abnormalities, abnormal facies, thymic hypoplasia, cleft palate, hypoparathyroid, chromosome 22

What are the clinical and laboratory manifestations of hyper-IgM syndrome?

Clinical: recurrent pyogenic bacterial infections early in life. Laboratory: see high IgM, but low IgG, IgA, IgE

What is the underlying genetic defect in hyper-IgM syndrome?

A mutation in CD40 ligand gene leads to a defective CD40L on T-cell surfaces. Without the proper CD40L-CD40 signaling, B cells cannot switch isotypes from IgM to other classes.

To what infections are patients with interleukin 12 (IL-12) receptor deficiency predisposed?

Disseminated mycobacterial infections, because IL-12 is involved in development of the cell-mediated Th1 response against mycobacteria

What types of immune cells are defective in severe combined immunodeficiency disease (SCID) and how is it inherited?	B and T cells. Most cases (75%) are X-linked.
How does SCID clinically manifest and how is it treated?	Patients are predisposed to recurrent bacterial, viral, fungal, and protozoal infections. Treat with bone marrow transplant.
What defects can lead to SCID?	Most common, about 50%, is the lack of the common γ chain of the IL-2, IL-4, IL-7, and IL-15 receptors (needed for T-cell development). The next most common is an adenosine deaminase (ADA) deficiency required for the purine salvage pathway.
How is Wiskott-Aldrich syndrome inherited and what is the classic triad of presentation?	X-linked recessive. Classic triad of eczema, recurrent infections, thrombocytopenia.
Which antibody isotypes levels are low in Wiskott-Aldrich syndrome? Which isotypes levels are high?	**IgE and IgM are high. IgG is normal or low and IgA is low**
What is the major defect in Wiskott-Aldrich syndrome and how is it treated?	Lack of an IgM response to bacterial capsules. Treat with bone marrow transplant.

Mnemonic:

1. Turn the **W** in **W**iskott upside down: **W** → Ig**M**
2. **X-PECT** (Expect) infections with Wiskott-Aldrich (**X**-linked, **P**yogenic infections, **C**apsular response impaired, **T**hrombocytopenia)

What cancer are patients with Wiskott-Aldrich syndrome prone to develop?	Non-Hodgkin lymphoma
How does ataxia-telangiectasia present?	Patients have recurrent infections at a young age in addition to uncoordinated gait (ataxia) and skin lesions consisting of small, dilated terminal vessels (telangiectasias)
How is ataxia-telangiectasia inherited and what is the genetic defect?	Autosomal recessive mutation in DNA repair enzymes
What immunoglobulin deficiency is often seen with ataxia-telangiectasia?	IgA deficiency

What is the genetic defect in chronic granulomatous disease (CGD) and how is it inherited?	Lack of nicotinamide adenine dinucleotide phosphate (NADPH) oxidase. Usually X-linked recessive
What are two diagnostic test for CGD?	Nitroblue-tetrazolium (NBT) and dihydrorhodamine flow cytometry. Failure to turn blue with NBT test and failure to produce rhodamine in DHT flow cytometry suggestive of CGD.
What is the function of NADPH oxidase and in what cells is it found?	NADPH oxidase helps generate H_2O_2 used in respiratory bursts of neutrophils.
What are the principal sources of infection in chronic CGD and the most common cause of death	Fungal and bacterial infections. Pneumonia due to *Aspergillus fumigatus* is the most common cause of death from chronic CGD.
What bacteria typically infect patients with CGD?	Catalase-positive bacteria (*Staphylococcus aureus* and *Escherichia coli*) that use catalase to degrade their endogenous H_2O_2. *Burkholderia cepacia* is the most common bacterial cause of death in CGD.
What bacteria can CGD patients resist?	Catalase-negative bacteria (*Streptococcus pyogenes*) that cannot degrade their endogenous H_2O_2, which is then utilized by neutrophils. The bacteria provide the bullet!
Chédiak-Higashi syndrome is due to a microtubule dysfunction, and presents with recurrent pyogenic infections. What are the two abnormalities seen in the immune cells of these patients?	1. Failure of lysosome/phagosome fusion → large granular inclusions of abnormal lysosomes 2. Abnormal neutrophil chemotaxis
What are the features of Job syndrome (hyper-IgE syndrome)?	High IgE, recurrent *cold* staphylococcal abscesses, eczema, and skeletal abnormalities
What is the underlying deficiency in Job syndrome?	Lack of γ-interferon (γ-IFN) production by Th1 cells (inflammatory cells)
What is a cold abscess?	Low γ-IFN favors the development of Th2 cells that are anti-inflammatory (and the source of IL-4 that induces B-cell production of IgE). Therefore, staphylococcal abscesses cannot trigger the *hot* or inflammatory response. **Mnemonic: GEt an EASy Job** (**G**amma-IFN, **I**gE, **E**czema, **A**bscesses, **S**keletal abnormalities)

What is leukocyte adhesion deficiency syndrome? How does it present? Which protein is defective in the most common type of leukocyte adhesion deficiency?

Autosomal recessive defect of lymphocyte function-associated antigen 1 (LFA-1), an adhesion protein on leukocytes, leads to severe pyogenic infections. CD18/integrin beta 2 is defective in type I leukocyte adhesion deficiency, the most common type. Essentially leukocytes cannot be brought to where they are needed.

Common variable immunodeficiency presents with recurrent pyogenic infections. What is the underlying cause of this disorder?

Hypogammaglobulinemia due to a block in B-cell differentiation to plasma cells

What immune cells are most affected in human immunodeficiency virus/acquired immunodeficiency syndrome (HIV/AIDS) and what types of immunity are compromised?

HIV targets CD4$^+$ helper T cells which results in dysfunction of both humoral and cell-mediated immunities.

What are some examples of bacterial infections that are common in AIDS patients?

Mycobacterium tuberculosis, Mycobacterium avium-complex, Streptococcus pneumoniae (most common case of pneumonia in AIDS patients, not PCP), *Salmonella*, etc.

What are some examples of viral infections that are common in AIDS patients?

Cytomegalovirus, papovavirus, JC virus, herpes simplex virus type 1 (HSV-1), varicella-zoster virus (VZV), Epstein-Barr virus (EBV)

What are some examples of fungal infections that are common in AIDS patients?

Cryptococcus, Candida, Histoplasma, Mucor, Pneumocystis jiroveci (formerly *Pneumocystis carinii*), *Coccidioides, Blastomyces*, etc.

What are some examples of protozoal infections that are common in AIDS patients?

Cryptosporidium, Toxoplasma, etc.

What infection are HIV$^+$ patients more susceptible to regardless of CD4 cell count?

Mycobacterium Tuberculosis

For what malignancies are AIDS patients at increased risk?

Kaposi sarcoma, Anal carcinoma, Non-Hodgkin lymphoma, and Cervical cancer **Mnemonic: (KANCer)**

CHAPTER 45

Laboratory Use of Antibodies

Describe the agglutination test to determine ABO blood type:

First, the sample blood is mixed separately with antiserum against both types A and B. Agglutination or clumping with antiserum suggests that the sample is of that blood group (no agglutination for type O).

Why does agglutination occur?

Extensive cross-linking between antigen-antibodies form complexes that result in agglutination.

Describe a precipitation test:

Increasing concentrations of antigen solution are plated in individual wells. A fixed amount of antibody is added to each well and the aggregation of antibody-antigen complexes are observed by visualization of precipitate.

What is the zone of equivalence in the antigen-precipitation technique?

The zone of equivalence is the solution of antigen concentration where the amount of antigen is approximately equivalent to antibody added. This equal proportion results in the largest amount of precipitate.

Explain how a sandwich enzyme-linked immunosorbent assay (ELISA) is performed:

1. Antibodies of known antigen specificity are coated on the sample plate.
2. Antigen containing sample of interest is added.
3. Excess antigen not bound to antibody is washed off.
4. Enzyme-linked antibodies, also of known antigen specificity, are added and the excess washed off.
5. Concentration of bound enzyme-linked antibody is determined by spectrometry when a color-changing substrate is added and acted upon by the antibody-linked enzyme.

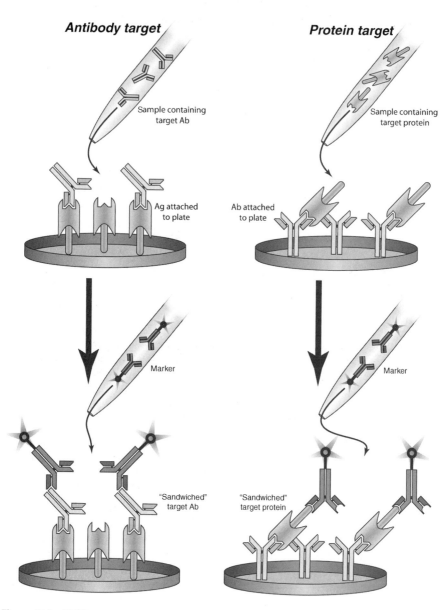

Antibody target

Sample containing target Ab

Ag attached to plate

Marker

"Sandwiched" target Ab

Protein target

Sample containing target protein

Ab attached to plate

Marker

"Sandwiched" target protein

Figure 45.1 ELISA.

How can the presence of an antibody be tested via ELISA?

The process is identical to identifying an antigen, but instead the antigen is coated to the sample plate and the sample containing the antibody in question is added to the antigen.

Is ELISA considered a direct or indirect antibody test?

ELISAs can be direct or indirect. A direct ELISA uses an enzyme-linked antibody specific for the antigen for detection. An indirect ELISA relies on identifying bound antigen-specific antibody with a second enzyme-linked antibody specific for the species of the primary antibody bound, which increases the sensitivity of the assay.

What is the conventional confirmatory test to determine the validity of screening ELISAs, such as those for human immunodeficiency virus (HIV) and Lyme disease?

Western blot

What are the key steps involved in a Western blot? Describe each step:

Gel electrophoresis: denatured/solubilized antigens are separated by molecular weight on gel by electrical current polarized positive to negative.

Transfer: antigens are transferred from the gel to a membrane by an electrical current polarized positive to negative (*photocopy* of the gel).

Antibody label: next a radioiodinated antibody specific for the antigen of interest is applied and binds antigen.

Autoradiography: the radio labeled membrane is exposed to x-ray film, resulting in the identification of an antigen as a darkened band on the film.

(Currently, most Western blots are performed with enzyme-linked antibodies, resulting in fluorescence which is exposed against x-ray film.)

Southern and Northern blot techniques are analogous to Western blots. What do Southern and Northern blots identify? What is used instead of radiolabeled antibody?

Southern blot identifies specific DNA sequences; Northern blot identifies specific RNA sequences. Both use DNA probes with radioactive phosphate that is complementary to the sequence of interest to be detected.

In a radioimmunoassay (RIA), an antigen-specific antibody competes for a known concentration of radiolabeled antigen and an unknown concentration of nonradiolabeled antigen. Next, the amount of radioactivity is measured, but what is needed to determine the unknown concentration?

A pregenerated standard curve of concentrations that correlates the amount of radioactivity measured to a final concentration of antigen

What is measured in the radioallergosorbent test (RAST)?

RAST is a specialized RIA in which the amount of serum immunoglobulin E (IgE) that reacts with a known allergen is quantified.

What is the primary purpose of using affinity chromatography on a serum sample?

Affinity chromatography allows a desired antigen to be separated from a mixture. The sample is run through a gel column with bound antibodies specific for the antigen. The sample is washed, while the antigen remains bound to the fixed antibodies, separating the desired molecule from the mixture.

In affinity chromatography, how is the desired antigen extracted from the bound antibodies?

A change in pH in the column buffer changes the charge and therefore binding affinities of the antibody and antigen, allowing the antigen to be eluted from the column.

In the complement fixation technique, an antigen of interest and patient's serum is mixed with complement. If addition of the sensitized red blood cells (RBCs) (RBC with the antigen of interest) results in hemolysis, what can be said about the result?

If the sensitized RBCs hemolyze, then it is a negative reaction. This implies that the patient's serum lacks the antibody to bind the antigen of interest. In a positive reaction, the sensitized RBCs do not hemolyze. This implies that the patient's serum have the specific antibody to bind the antigen of interest. The antibody-antigen complex then activates the complement so that when sensitized RBCs are added to the mixture, there is no complement left to hemolyze the RBCs.

Limulus amoebocyte lysate (LAL) is a purified extract from the horseshoe crabs that is used to test the sterility of surgical equipment. Upon exposure to endotoxin from gram-negative bacteria, LAL will rapidly clump together, indicating contaminated equipment. What type of test is this best characterized as?

Active hemagglutination

What is the difference between passive and active hemagglutination?

Active hemagglutination results from the clumping of native blood cells in response to antigen impurities such as viruses. By contrast, passive hemagglutination requires the blood cells to first passively absorb antigens (e.g., viral antigens) from solution, and then clump upon administration of antibodies specific for the antigen.

What is the difference in the target of detection between the direct and indirect versions of the Coombs test?

The Coombs test is an agglutination test that detects anti-RBC antibodies. Direct Coombs tests attempts to detect antibodies attached on the RBCs. Indirect Coombs test attempts to detect antibodies in the serum.

How are cells identified in flow cytometry?

Cells are *tagged* with fluorescently labeled antibodies to various surface markers (e.g., CD4, CD8). A laser then detects the wavelength of light emitted from each fluorescent antibody (red vs green) and records the number of times that wavelength was encountered. Cells may be not labeled, labeled by only one fluorescent antibody, or by multiple fluorescent antibodies.

How are cells sorted in flow cytometry?

A fluorescence-activated cell sorter (FACS) separates cells by the electromagnetic charges applied to the fluorescent signals. Cells with no fluorescence, only one fluorescent antibody, or multiple fluorescent antibodies are deflected (and thus sorted) differently.

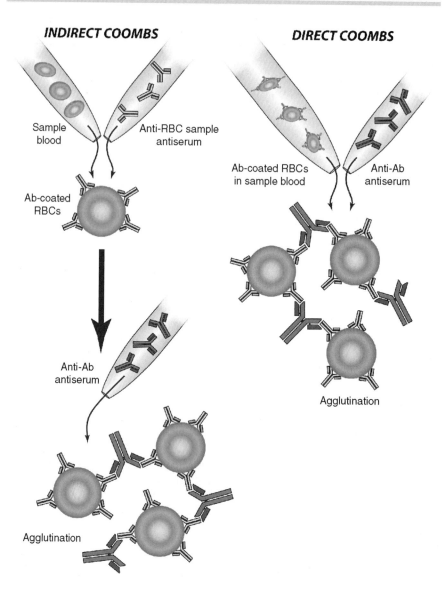

Figure 45.2   Coombs test.

Systems-Based Microbiology

CHAPTER 46

Cardiovascular System

What components of the cardiovascular system are prone to infections? Name each type of infection:	Myocardium (myocarditis), pericardium (pericarditis), endocardium (endocarditis), blood (sepsis), and blood vessels (thrombophlebitis or endarteritis)

MYOCARDITIS

Is myocarditis a common disease?	No, it is quite rare.
What commonly precedes the symptoms of viral myocarditis?	Flu-like illness (fever, malaise, myalgia) 1 to 2 weeks prior to symptoms of myocarditis that spontaneously resolved
What are some symptoms of acute myocarditis?	Fatigue, palpitations, dyspnea, pulmonary rales, S3 gallop, chest pain, cardiogenic shock, arrhythmias
What other conditions are related in a differential diagnosis of myocarditis?	Acute coronary syndrome, pericarditis, congestive heart failure (CHF)
What are the most common viral causes of myocarditis?	Coxsackievirus B (most common), human immunodeficiency virus (HIV), echovirus, adenovirus type 2, influenza virus, hepatitis C, and cytomegalovirus (CMV)
Which infections cause myocarditis in the immunocompromised?	Toxoplasmosis and cytomegalovirus commonly have no symptoms until immune system is compromised from a neoplasm, HIV, or a transplant.
When is the peak time of year for Coxsackie infections?	Summer and early fall

What are some common nonviral, infectious causes of myocarditis?

Numerous causes including *Rickettsia rickettsii* (Rocky Mountain spotted fever [RMSF]), *Borrelia burgdorferi* (Lyme disease), syphilis, *Trypanosoma cruzi* (Chagas disease), *Toxoplasma*, and many fungi

When treating a patient with *Rickettsia*, what antibiotic is used for patients with renal insufficiency?

Doxycycline over tetracycline due to doxy being excreted by the liver

What is the name of the reaction that tests positive for RMSF that uses the *Proteus* antigen?

Weil-Felix reaction is an assay for antirickettsial antibodies that cross-react with *Proteus*.

What are other important cardiac problems caused by *B. burgdorferi* infection?

Arrhythmia (atrioventricular conduction delay) and pericarditis commonly 1 week but up to 1 to 2 months after infection

What is the most common parasitic cause of heart failure in the world?

Heart failure secondary to cardiomegaly from *Trypanosoma cruzi* (Chagas disease) infection

What is the predominate cell type infiltrate present in viral myocarditis?

Lymphocytes

Which upper respiratory infectious bacteria can cause myocarditis?

Corynebacterium diphtheriae

PERICARDITIS

What is acute pericarditis?

Inflammation of the pericardium, which can be classified as fibrinous (dry) or effusive (serous or hemorrhagic)

What are some clinical signs and symptoms of acute pericarditis?

Pericardial friction rub, sharp retrosternal pain worse on inspiration and supine position, better leaning forward. Pain commonly radiates to shoulders (phrenic nerve supplies both), high or spiking fever (helps differentiate from noninfectious cause).

What is a friction rub?

High-pitched, scratching, grating sound most frequently heard in systole when the patient is exhaling in the sitting position. Best heard when applying pressure at the left lower sternal border

What is the diagnostic sign on an electrocardiogram (ECG)?

Diffuse ST elevations

Name the most common viral causes of pericarditis:

Human immunodeficiency virus (HIV), Coxsackievirus A and B, echovirus, mumps, adenovirus, and hepatitis

Name the other common causes of pericarditis:

Tuberculosis (more common in developing countries), staphylococcal or pneumococcal infection (pyogenic), amebiasis, actinomycosis, and fungi

What bacteria is associated with long-term autoimmune-mediated pericarditis?

Streptococcus pyogenes (strep throat)

What are the long-term complications of acute pericarditis?

Cardiac tamponade, constrictive pericarditis

What are the common noninfectious causes of pericarditis?

Post-MI inflammation (acute, and Dressler syndrome), neoplasm, uremia, autoimmune disorders (systemic lupus erythematosus [SLE], etc)

ENDOCARDITIS

What are some clinical signs and symptoms of infectious endocarditis?

Commonly fevers, chills, malaise. Also present with Janeway lesions (pathognomic, embolized microabscesses in dermis of hands or feet), Osler nodes (nonspecific, painful, immune complex deposition), splinter hemorrhages, Roth spots (nonspecific retinal hemorrhage with pale, fibrin center), new-onset murmur, CHF

What is the name of the criteria set for diagnosing infective endocarditis?

Duke criteria

What valve is most commonly infected in infectious endocarditis? Second most common?

Mitral valve. Second most common is aortic valve.

How is endocarditis diagnosed?

Transthoracic or transesophageal echocardiogram (ultrasound of heart) to look for vegetations (mass of fibrin, thrombus, platelet, bacteria), three sets of blood cultures spaced an hour apart, and history/physical examination

What species of bacteria is the most common cause of acute infectious endocarditis?

Staphylococcus aureus from skin flora

What group of bacteria is the most common cause of subacute infectious endocarditis?

Viridans group streptococci from oral flora

What other groups of bacteria are clinically significant causes of endocarditis?

Staphylococci and streptococci (including coagulase-negative staphylococci, enterococci, etc) cause more than 80% of all endocarditis. The HACEK (*Haemophilus aphrophilus, Actinobacillus actinomycetemcomitans, Cardiobacterium hominis, Eikenella corrodens,* and *Kingella kingae*) respiratory flora group causes about 2%

What cancer and which bacteria have been found to be associated with endocarditis?

Colon cancer and *Streptococcus gallolyticus*

What is the difference between acute and subacute infectious endocarditis?

Acute infectious endocarditis is characterized by infection with highly virulent *S. aureus* and large vegetations on the valve with significant valvular destruction and the potential to embolize. Subacute infectious endocarditis, while also fatal if untreated, typically is caused by Viridans group streptococci and usually forms small vegetations on damaged or prosthetic valves and has a more gradual onset.

Intravenous (IV) drug abuse increases the risk of what type of endocarditis? What species of bacteria is usually involved and which valve is classically damaged?

Acute infectious endocarditis by *S. aureus*; it is classically associated with damage to the tricuspid valve (bacteria from vein reach tricuspid first)

Which fungal endocarditis is particularly common in IV drug users?

Candida albicans

What are some other risk factors associated with endocarditis?

History of rheumatic fever (remember to always ask patients with new-onset murmurs), congenital valve problems, and prosthetic valves (bacteria tend to adhere to damaged valves)

What common congenital valve conditions predispose patients to endocarditis, especially after invasive dental procedures?

Bicuspid aortic valve and mitral valve prolapse (a common condition especially in young women). Invasive dental procedures cause transient bacteremia especially with Viridans group *Streptococcus.*

What are some daily activities that can cause bacteremia?

Brushing teeth, defecation, and tongue bites. Patients who don't floss are slightly higher risk for infectious endocarditis.

What species of bacteria causes endocarditis after procedures related to the gastrointestinal (GI) or genitourinary (GU) tract?

Enterococcus faecalis

What is the common antibiotic combination treatment for subacute endocarditis?

Penicillin with aminoglycoside. Prior to antibiotic therapy almost all patients with infectious endocarditis died; now more than 80% survive.

What characteristic of bacterial growth makes endocarditis difficult to treat?

Biofilm formation by dextran by Viridans group *Streptococcus* or coagulase-negative *Staphylococcus*

What organs are commonly affected by infective emboli?

Brain (causing stroke, meningitis), spleen (septic infarct), joint (septic), kidneys (urinary tract infection [UTI]), lungs (septic infarct)

What is in a differential diagnosis of infective endocarditis?

Rheumatic fever, atrial myxoma, Libman-Sacks endocarditis, nonbacterial thrombotic endocarditis (marantic)

BLOOD AND VESSEL-RELATED INFECTIONS

What bacteria are normally found in human blood?

None! Normally human blood is free of microbes.

What is the difference between bacteremia, systemic inflammatory response syndrome (SIRS), sepsis, severe sepsis, and septic shock?

Bacteremia is the presence of bacteria in the blood. SIRS is a systemic inflammatory response with two of the following four conditions: temperature (>38°C or <36°C), heart rate (>90 beats/min), respiratory rate (>20 breaths/min) or Paco2 (<32 mm Hg), white blood cell (WBC) (>12,000 cells/mm3). Sepsis is SIRS plus known source of infection. Severe sepsis is sepsis plus end organ damage. Septic shock is severe sepsis plus hypotension.

What is commonly the source of persistent bacteremia?	Infectious endocarditis

What infectious etiologies cause the following types of anemia:

Megaloblastic anemia	Vitamin B12 deficiency caused by *Diphyllobothrium latum* (freshwater fish tapeworm common in Great Lakes region among other locations)
Microcytic anemia	Iron deficiency caused by hookworm (*Ancylostoma* or *Necator*) uncommon in the United States. Also may be secondary to blood loss from peptic ulcers related to *H. pylori*.
Normocytic anemia	Anemia of chronic disease by chronic infections (e.g., tuberculosis [TB], HIV, and the like)
Aplastic crisis	Parvovirus B19 in the setting of congenital hemolytic anemia (sickle cell, hereditary spherocytosis)
Hemolytic anemia	Infections associated with disseminated intravascular coagulation (DIC), thrombotic thrombocytopenic purpura-hemolytic uremic syndrome (TTP-HUS), malaria, or *Babesia*
What parasitic infection causes decreased hemoglobin and hematocrit with cyclical fevers?	*Plasmodium* (malaria)
Which intraerythrocytic bacterium is associated with *Borrelia burgdorferi*?	*Babesia microti* is found to be coinfected commonly with *Borrelia*. They are transmitted both by the hard tick *Ixodes*. Babesias form a "maltese cross" which is diagnostic inside of erythrocytes. **Mnemonic:** Ixotic BaBE (*Ehrlichia* is also transmitted by *Ixodes*)
What virus is classically associated with lymphocytosis and atypical lymphocytes?	Epstein-Barr virus (EBV) causes atypical T lymphocytes to react to infected B lymphocytes.
What parasites cause eosinophilia?	Helminths during migration through tissue. Common with schistosomiasis among others

What is septic (or supportive) thrombophlebitis?

A serious inflammatory condition in which suppuration occurs within the vein wall, subsequently causing thrombus and pus to form within the vein's lumen leading to perivascular inflammation and purulence

What are the most common causes of septic thrombophlebitis?

Staphylococcus aureus and *Streptococcus* species

What type of cells does *Rickettsia* preferentially infect?

Endothelial cells causing vasculitis and the characteristic rash

How is aortitis caused by *Treponema pallidum* tertiary syphilis classically described?

Tree-bark appearance in the ascending aorta

What bacteria can mimic Kaposi sarcoma in immunocompromised patients?

Bartonella—bacillary angiomatosis can cause nodular, red-/purple-colored vascular cutaneous lesions by angiogenesis and neutrophil inflammation. Both *Bartonella henselae* (cat scratch disease) and *Bartonella quintana* (body lice) are associated.

Which mosquito-borne disease is associated with spontaneous GI bleeding after being infected a second time?

Dengue fever (*flavivirus*) is associated with hemorrhagic fever or shock syndrome on reinfection with a different serotype.

Which mold proliferates in blood vessel walls causing infarction to distal tissue?

Mucor and *Rhizopus*. Nonseptate hyphae that particularly affect paranasal sinuses, lungs, or gut. Patients with diabetic ketoacidosis, burns, or leukemia are more susceptible.

OTHER HEART DISEASE

What is rheumatic heart disease?

Feared and most serious complication of rheumatic fever following S. *pyogenes* infection. Patients develop a whole host of heart diseases such as pancarditis, valve insufficiency and damage, arrhythmias, and ventricular dysfunction.

What are some distinguishing biochemical characteristics of S. *pyogenes*?

Produces large zone of β-hemolysis, pyrrolidonyl aminopeptidase (PYR) positive, susceptible to bacitracin

How does *S. pyogenes* cause rheumatic fever and/or rheumatic heart disease?

While the exact pathogenesis is unknown, molecular mimicry is thought to play a role leading to autoimmune damage.

Which virus is associated with cardiomyopathy and the immunocompromised?

HIV virus has been associated with direct cardiomyopathy, even independent of opportunistic infections. Cardiac involvement is varied but occurs later in the disease as CD4 counts fall.

By which parasitic organism is Cysticercosis of the heart caused?

Taenia solium (pork tapeworm), ingestion of the larva form

***Trypanosoma cruzi* causes Chagas disease, which causes megaesophagus, megacolon, and Chagas heart disease. What are the main symptoms of Chagas heart disease?**

Heart failure, heart block, malignant arrhythmias, and thromboembolism

CHAPTER 47

Respiratory System

ORAL AND NASAL CAVITY

What are the most prevalent species of bacteria in the mouth?	Viridans group streptococci, particularly *Streptococcus mutans*
Why must patients with valvular heart damage be placed on prophylactic antibiotics when undergoing dental work?	Transient bacteremia occurs during dental work that raises the risk for subacute endocarditis. Prophylactic antibiotics no longer recommended for mitral valve prolapse.
Name at least three normal bacterial floras of the gingival crevices that can cause a lung abscess if aspirated, especially in debilitated patients:	1. *Bacteroides* 2. *Fusobacterium* 3. *Peptostreptococcus* 4. *Actinomyces israelii*
What radiographic finding is present for a lung abscess?	Air-fluid levels
What predisposing factors cause an increased risk of aspiration?	Esophageal dysmotility, seizure disorders, periodontal disease, dementia, impaired consciousness, and alcoholism
What fungus, which is part of normal flora, causes thrush in immunocompromised patients?	*Candida albicans*
How can oral thrush be diagnosed?	Potassium hydroxide (KOH) scrapings to look for pseudohyphae and buds. Some forms of candidiasis cannot be scraped off (hyperplastic); such forms can resemble leukoplakia.
What virus is associated with white, frond-like lesions along the lateral portions of the tongue in human immunodeficiency virus (HIV)-positive patients?	Epstein-Barr virus (EBV) causing oral hairy leukoplakia. Represents an advanced immunological decline

Name the condition associated with dark, purple lesions in the oral cavity of HIV-positive patients:

Kaposi sarcoma—a neoplastic collection of vasculature. Must also rule out lymphoma

Name the virus class and condition associated with painful lesions in the oral cavity, on the hands, and on the feet:

Enterovirus (most common Coxsackie)— hand-foot-mouth disease (HFMD). HFMD is common in infants and children and is very contagious.

Name the virus associated with painful oral vesicles following 2- to 3-day prodrome that eventually ulcerates:

Herpes simplex virus (HSV) causing HSV stomatitis commonly located around oral mucosa, tongue, palate, vermillion border, and gingiva

What infectious disease and virus is associated with Koplik spots?

Rubeola (measles) virus is associated with red spots with blue-white center on buccal mucosa. Also found with three C's: cough, coryza (head cold), and conjunctivitis along with rash spreading from head to toe. Long-term risk of SSPE (subacute sclerosing panencephalitis)

Which bacteria cause honey-crusted lesions common in children in near the mouth?

Impetigo, an infectious skin condition common in kids in the perioral and nasal areas, is caused by *Staphylococcus aureus* (most commonly), and group A streptococci.

What two fungi are important causes of necrotizing sinusitis, especially in the immunocompromised?

1. *Aspergillus*
2. Zygomycetes (especially *Mucor* and *Rhizopus*)

What specific conditions are *Mucor* and *Rhizopus* associated with?

Diabetic ketoacidosis, burns, leukemia. Molds proliferate in blood vessel walls and cause infarcts of supplied tissue.

Name two important gram-positive organisms that normally colonize the nose:

Streptococcus and *Staphylococcus* species, particularly *S. aureus*

Which virus is the most frequent cause of the common cold and has more than 100 antigenic subtypes?

Rhinoviruses (peaks during spring and fall). Preferentially grow at 33°C to 34°C which is the temperature of the nasal passages

Which other viruses also cause the common cold syndrome?

Coronavirus (winter-spring), adenovirus, influenza C virus, and Coxsackievirus

PHARYNX

What is the most common cause of pharyngitis (sore throat)?	Viruses such as rhinoviruses or coronaviruses
Why should aspirin never be used to treat fever in children?	Feared complication of Reye syndrome (encephalopathy, liver failure) when aspirin is used in children with influenza or chickenpox
What is the most common cause of exudative bacterial pharyngitis with fever, cervical lymphadenopathy, and leukocytosis?	*Streptococcus pyogenes*
What laboratory features allow for the diagnosis of S. *pyogenes*?	Colonies are catalase-negative, β-hemolytic, and bacitracin-sensitive (inhibited by bacitracin disk). Elevated antistreptolysin (ASO) or anti-DNAse B titer indicates prior infection.
Why should S. *pyogenes* pharyngitis be treated if it usually spontaneously resolves?	Untreated S. *pyogenes* infections may extend to otitis, sinusitis, mastoiditis, and meningitis, and may lead to immune-mediated complications, including acute glomerulonephritis and acute rheumatic fever.
What type of glomerulonephritis is a streptococcal infection associated with? What is the most common urinary complaint?	Nephritic syndrome (hematuria, hypertension [HTN], oliguria, azotemia)—acute poststreptococcal glomerulonephritis represented by subepithelial humps on electron microscopy and granular pattern on immunofluorescence. Commonly presents 2 weeks after initial infection with complaint of "tea/cola colored urine."
What is the standard treatment of S. *pyogenes* pharyngitis?	Penicillin G or a macrolide if allergic
Which species of bacteria causes membranous pharyngitis associated with a low-grade fever, obstructive laryngotracheitis, and *bull neck* from cervical adenopathy?	*Corynebacterium diphtheriae*
What is the mechanism of action of its exotoxin?	Inhibits protein synthesis by adenosine diphosphate (ADP) ribosylation of elongation factor 2 (EF-2)

How does a strain of *C. diphtheriae* gain the exotoxin?	β-Prophage infection with encoded toxin
Name three serious complications of *C. diphtheriae* infection:	1. Obstructive laryngotracheitis (extension of the membrane into the larynx and trachea causing airway obstruction) 2. Myocarditis (abnormal electrocardiogram [ECG]) 3. Neuropathy
What is the treatment of *C. diphtheriae* infection?	Diphtheria equine antitoxin, removal of the membrane by direct laryngoscope or bronchoscopy, antibiotic therapy (penicillin, erythromycin, azithromycin, clarithromycin), and isolation of the patient until cultures at the completion of treatment document elimination of the organism from the oropharynx
How is *C. diphtheriae* infection prevented?	Active immunization with diphtheria toxoid as part of routine childhood immunization (usually as diphtheria and tetanus toxoids and acellular pertussis [DTaP]) with appropriate booster injections. Forms antibodies to B subunit of exotoxin
What type of patient population is diphtheria common in? How does it present? How is it identified?	Immigrants without any immunization therapy. Presents with neuropathy, paralysis, or heart failure. Diagnosis based on staining of club-shaped, gram-positive rods with metachromatic granules and ELEK test (used to determine whether the cultured *C. diphtheriae* contains the toxin encoding phage)
What organism typically infects young children and is characterized by a high-pitched inspiratory *whoop* and lymphocytosis?	*Bordetella pertussis*
How is *B. pertussis* cultured to confirm diagnosis?	Specimen from a nasopharyngeal swab taken during the paroxysmal stage and grown on Bordet-Gengou agar
How does *B. pertussis* attach to the respiratory epithelium?	Via a protein on the pili called filamentous hemagglutinin

Briefly describe the pertussis toxin's effect on adenylate cyclase:	Inactivates G_i via ADP ribosylation, causing a rise in cyclic adenosine monophosphate (cAMP) and downstream cAMP-dependent protein kinase activity
What endocrine organ is affected by the pertussis toxin?	Islet cells can be activated and cause resulting hypoglycemia.
How does *B. pertussis* present in adults?	It is less severe but prolonged (100-day cough), and the characteristic *whoop* may be absent.
How is *B. pertussis* infection prevented? Treated?	Active immunization with pertussis toxin as part of routine childhood immunization (usually as DTaP) with follow-up booster vaccine with tetanus toxoid, reduced diphtheria toxoid, and acellular pertussis (Tdap) which forms immunoglobulin A (IgA) antibodies. Treated with macrolides, preferably azithromycin and clarithromycin.
What virus causes pharyngitis associated with severe fatigue, lymphadenopathy, lymphocytosis, fever, and rash?	Epstein-Barr virus (mono) (also cytomegalovirus [CMV], human immunodeficiency virus [HIV])
If a patient, not allergic to penicillin, breaks out in a rash after being treated with penicillin for suspected streptococcal pharyngitis, what should you think?	Epstein-Barr viral pharyngitis
What would a complete blood count (CBC) and blood smear show in Epstein-Barr virus (EBV) infection?	CBC demonstrating leukocytosis with absolute lymphocytosis and peripheral blood smear demonstrating atypical T lymphocytes that are large and have lobulated nuclei
What does the monospot test look for?	Heterophile antibodies that can agglutinate sheep RBCs.
What cancers are associated with EBV?	Burkitt lymphoma and other B-cell lymphomas, nasopharyngeal carcinoma, oral hairy leukoplakia, and central nervous system (CNS) lymphoma in AIDS patients
What virus is associated with hand-foot-mouth syndrome and herpangina, a painful vesicular blister of the mouth?	Coxsackie A

LARYNX

Which virus is the leading cause of croup (acute laryngotracheobronchitis) in young children and is an important cause of the common cold in adults?

Parainfluenza virus

Though far less common, which bacterium is associated with laryngitis?

Group A streptococci

EPIGLOTTIS

How severe is epiglottitis? Why is it not a common problem?

Acute epiglottitis is a medical emergency due to possibility of compromised airway. Because of vaccination with the *Haemophilus influenzae* type B (Hib) vaccine, rates of infection have fallen.

How does a patient present with acute epiglottitis?

Respiratory obstruction, dyspnea, drooling, stridor, sore throat, systemic toxicity, high fever. Oropharynx will commonly appear less severe than symptoms.

What is the "thumbprint sign" seen on neck radiograph?

Edematous epiglottis seen on lateral neck films

What bacterium is an important cause of epiglottitis, meningitis, and sepsis in children and causes pneumonia in adults, particularly in those with chronic obstructive pulmonary disease (COPD)?

Haemophilus influenzae with capsular type B responsible for most invasive diseases

What is the culture medium requirement to isolate *H. influenzae*?

Heated blood (*chocolate*) agar enriched with growth factors V (nicotinamide adenine dinucleotide [NAD]) and X (hematin)

Does *H. influenzae* type B (Hib) vaccine protect against *H. influenzae* epiglottitis and meningitis?

Yes, but it does **not** protect against *H. influenzae* otitis media, bronchitis, and pneumonia tag. Note that Hib protects against all infections of *H. influenzae* type B but not nontypeable *H. influenzae* infections.

What is the appropriate chemoprophylactic for individuals exposed to sick contacts with *H. influenzae* type B?

Rifampin

BRONCHUS

What is the most common presentation of acute bronchitis?

Cough (not caused by pneumonia or chronic bronchitis) for less than 1 or 2 weeks

What is the most common cause of acute bronchitis?

Viral: influenza A and B, parainfluenza, respiratory syncytial virus (RSV)

Which virus is the most common cause of bronchiolitis in children?

Respiratory syncytial virus

What are the most common causes of bacterial bronchitis?

Mycoplasma pneumoniae, Chlamydia pneumoniae, B. pertussis, and *Legionella*

What are the most common causes of acute exacerbation of chronic bronchitis (AECB)?

Bacterial: *H. influenzae, S. pneumoniae*, and *Moraxella catarrhalis*

What characterizes AECB?

Increased dyspnea, increased cough and sputum production, and increasing purulence of sputum. Common in COPD patients, elderly, diminished lung function, or those with chronic steroid use

LUNGS

What are the most common causes of bacterial pneumonia in neonates?

Group B streptococci, *Escherichia coli*

What are the common infectious causes of subacute/chronic cough that can resemble an upper respiratory infection (URI) or pneumonia?

Viral (influenza, RSV, parainfluenza), *M. pneumoniae, C. pneumoniae, B. pertussis, Legionella*, coccidioidomycosis

What is the most common cause of bacterial pneumonia in teenagers and young adults?

Mycoplasma pneumoniae

What are typical symptoms of *M. pneumoniae* pneumonia?

Gradual onset of fever, sore throat, malaise, and a persistent dry, hacking cough. Chills and tachycardia are uncommon.

What are the classic findings on a chest x-ray (CXR) for *M. pneumoniae* infection?

Prominent streaky infiltrate, which usually looks worse than the clinical and physical examinations suggest

What are cold agglutinins and how are they used to diagnose *M. pneumoniae* infection?

Antibodies against type O red blood cells that agglutinate these cells at 4°C but not at 37°C. A cold agglutinin titer of more than 1:128 indicates recent *M. pneumoniae* infection.

Can penicillins or cephalosporins be used to treat *M. pneumoniae* infections?

No, *M. pneumoniae* has no cell wall.

What is atypical pneumonia? What organisms cause atypical pneumonia?

Atypical pneumonia technically refers to pneumonias that do not resemble *pneumococcal* pneumonia in clinical presentation, diagnosis, and treatment. Atypical pneumonias include *M. pneumoniae* (most common), *Legionella pneumophila, C. pneumoniae, Chlamydia psittaci, Francisella tularensis, Mycobacterium tuberculosis, Coxiella burnetii*, and viral pneumonias.

What is the difference between atypical pneumonia and walking pneumonia?

Do not confuse atypical pneumonia with *walking* pneumonia (though the two are often used interchangeably). Walking pneumonia often refers to pneumonia with low-grade fever, mild-to-moderate symptoms (hospitalization not needed), and an interstitial infiltrate. Recall, even though *M. pneumoniae* and *C. pneumoniae* do result in interstitial infiltrate, *L. pneumophila* causes a lobar pneumonia.

Which species of bacteria causes atypical pneumonia and hepatitis in patients with a history of bird exposure?

Chlamydia psittaci

Which species of bacteria causes a mild flu-like illness, pneumonia, and hepatitis in patients with exposure to the placental products of farm animals?

Coxiella burnetii (Q fever)

Which organism is the most common cause of lobar pneumonia, otitis media, and sinusitis?

Streptococcus pneumoniae

Describe the classic clinical presentation and chest x-ray findings in a patient with _S. pneumoniae_ pneumonia:

Sudden onset of chills, fever, pleuritic chest pain, and a cough productive of blood-tinged (_rusty_) sputum. Chest x-ray demonstrating lobar consolidation with air bronchograms

What are the findings on blood agar for _S. pneumoniae_?

Small α-hemolytic colonies that are bile-soluble and growth is inhibited by optochin.

What is the most important virulence factor of _S. pneumoniae_?

Capsular polysaccharide. Anticapsular antibody (induced by the vaccine) is protective.

What virulence factor of _S. pneumoniae_ is shared with _H. influenzae_ and facilitates their attachment to the respiratory epithelium?

Immunoglobulin A (IgA) protease that degrades secretory IgA allowing them to attach to and colonize mucosal surfaces

Name three species of encapsulated bacteria that can cause respiratory tract infections:

1. _Streptococcus pneumoniae_
2. _Haemophilus influenzae_
3. _Klebsiella pneumoniae_

Mnemonic: Capsules **P**rotect **N**aughty **H**uman **K**illing **S**trains of bacteria (_**C**ryptococcus neoformans_, _**P**seudomonas_, _**N**eisseria meningitidis_, _**H**. influenzae_, _**K**lebsiella_, _**S**treptococcus pneumoniae_).

What test can be used to differentiate encapsulated organisms from the many other causes of respiratory infections?

Quellung reaction

Name the organisms that most commonly cause hospital-acquired (nosocomial) pneumonia:

Pseudomonas aeruginosa, _S. aureus_, _Enterobacter_, _K. pneumoniae_, and _E. coli_

What bacterium is associated with causing infections in burn, neutropenic, and cystic fibrosis patients?

Pseudomonas aeruginosa

What gives _Pseudomonas_ colonies their distinguished color?

Pyocyanin gives them a blue-green color.

What is the mechanism of action of the _Pseudomonas_ toxin?

ADP ribosylates EF-2 to inhibit protein synthesis, similar to diphtheria toxin

What are the risk factors for _P. aeruginosa_?

Bronchiectasis, corticosteroid therapy, recent antibiotic therapy, malnutrition, and cystic fibrosis, diabetes

What is the common radiographic finding of bronchiectasis?	"Tramlines" which are parallel line shadows on CXR
What is a common cause of pneumonia in alcoholics, diabetics, or chronic obstructive pulmonary disease (COPD) patients that produces a red currant jelly-like sputum?	*Klebsiella pneumoniae*
What are the biochemical characteristics of *K. pneumoniae*?	Oxidase-negative, lactose-fermenting, gram-negative rod with a large polysaccharide capsule
What type of bacteria classically cause *a foul-smelling* pneumonia from aspiration?	Anaerobic bacteria
Name three gram-negative rods that commonly cause respiratory tract infections:	1. *Haemophilus* 2. *Legionella* 3. *Bordetella*
What is a major risk factor for gram-negative rod pneumonia?	Long-term care facilities or nursing home residents
What are some risk factors associated with *L. pneumophila* infections and how is the organism transmitted?	History of tobacco use, alcohol, and immunosuppression. It is transmitted from water sources such as humidifiers or air conditioners. There is no person-to-person transmission.
What other organ system complaint is common with a *Legionella* infection?	Gastrointestinal upset, diarrhea
What is a simple test to diagnose *Legionella* that is unique?	Urinary antigen screen can detect *Legionella*; however, the antigen remains positive for weeks even after treatment has been started and only identifies one serogroup.
What stain is required to identify *Legionella*?	Silver impregnated stain or direct fluorescent antibody (DFA) stain since it Gram stains poorly
What special medium is required to culture *Legionella*?	Charcoal yeast extract supplemented with iron and cysteine
What empiric antibiotic treatment can be used for *L. pneumophila*, *M. pneumoniae*, and *S. pneumoniae* (community-acquired pneumonia)?	Erythromycin or azithromycin (with or without rifampin) or fluoroquinolones

How does *Legionella* infection present?	Legionnaires' disease (severe pneumonia, fever, GI upset, CNS involvement, and hyponatremia) and Pontiac fever (mild flu-like symptoms).
What are some life-threatening complications that may arise from inhalation of *Bacillus anthracis* spores?	Hemorrhagic mediastinitis, bloody pleural effusions, and septic shock
What lipid is only found in acid-fast organisms and is involved in the virulence of *Mycobacterium*?	Mycolic acid, a large fatty acid
What are the symptoms of tuberculosis (TB)?	Fever, night sweats, weight loss, and hemoptysis.
What symptoms can TB mimic?	Lymphoma B—symptoms (fever, night sweats, weight loss), *Aspergillus* infection (insidious hemoptysis)
What is the cell wall structure that causes serpentine growth and inhibits leukocyte migration and killing?	Cord factor (trehalose)
Acid-fast staining is also known as:	Ziehl-Neelsen stain
Which staining method uses fluorescence microscopy?	Auramine-rhodamine stain
Why is sputum culturing for TB not of great value?	*Mycobacterium* has a slow growth rate and can take longer than 6 weeks to get a useful result. Lowenstein-Jensen agar is used.
Name key factors associated with an increased risk of reactivation of tuberculosis:	HIV infection or any medical condition leading to immunosuppression, persons who have converted their purified protein derivative (PPD) skin test in the past 2 years
What type of immune reaction occurs to result in a positive PPD test for tuberculosis?	Delayed-type (type IV) hypersensitivity reaction
When is a PPD test positive?	Patients with active infections (some patients only, and PPD is not used to diagnose active tuberculosis [TB]), latent infections, previously treated infections, and previous immunization with bacillus Calmette-Guérin (BCG) vaccine (although PPD reactivity declines with time). Induration must be 15 mm or more in a healthy person to be positive. 10 mm or more in individuals with high risk to TB exposure such as health-care workers. 5 mm or more in HIV-positive and immunocompromised individuals.

When is a PPD test negative?

If there has been no prior infection or there is anergy commonly from advanced HIV, steroids, malnutrition, sarcoidosis, or other immunocompromised state

In what part of the lungs does primary TB tend to develop?

The areas that receive the highest airflow and the middle and lower lung zones

In what part of the lungs does secondary reactivated TB tend to develop?

Apical areas because this is where oxygen tension is highest and *M. tuberculosis* is an aerobic bacterium

What is the name for a calcified tubercle in the middle or lower lung zone?

Ghon focus

What is the name of a Ghon focus accompanied by perihilar lymph node calcifications?

Ghon complex. Macrophages carrying the bacteria are transported from focus to lymph nodes to form a complex, unable to kill bacterium due to mycobacteria's preventing fusion of phagosome with lysosome and acidification of phagosome.

What is the most common site of reactivation tuberculosis?

Lungs, in the posterior apical segments, leading to pulmonary tuberculosis

What other body sites are locations for reactivation tuberculosis?

Bones, vertebral body (Pott disease), brain, meninges, genitourinary (GU) tract, and gastrointestinal (GI) tract

Name the most common causes of viral pneumonia in immunocompromised patients:

Cytomegalovirus (especially common in posttransplant patients), varicella-zoster virus, adenovirus, influenza, parainfluenza

Which highly infectious virus is associated with lymphopenia and an elevated lactate dehydrogenase (LDH)?

Severe acute respiratory syndrome (SARS) virus (coronavirus)

What respiratory complications can the measles virus, known for the maculopapular (morbilliform) rash and Koplik spots, also potentially cause?

Primary giant-cell pneumonia and secondary bacterial pneumonia

What virus causes pneumonia, myalgias, sore throat, cough, and is a significant cause of death in the elderly?

Influenza virus

Which viral pneumonia is acquired by direct contact or inhalation of rodent urine or feces?

Hantavirus can cause respiratory failure from edema or myocardial failure.

Name some common causes of fungal pneumonia in immunocompromised patients:

Aspergillus, Mucor, Histoplasma Coccidioides, Blastomyces

What are the important morphological characteristics of *Aspergillus*?

Exists only as mold (nondimorphic), has septate hyphae that form V-shaped (dichotomous) branches with parallel walls, and conidia radiating in chains

What are the main forms of *Aspergillus* infections?

Allergic bronchopulmonary aspergillosis (ABPA), aspergilloma, invasive aspergillosis.

What conditions predispose to

Cystic fibrosis, burns, chronic

***Aspergillus* infections?**

granulomatous disease (neutrophils can't properly kill fungus)

What is ABPA? What serum antibody is elevated in ABPA?

ABPA is a noninvasive infection of *Aspergillus fumigatus* that leads to type I hypersensitivity, and airway hyperreactivity. Usually occurs in asthmatics. IgE is elevated. Patients will expectorate brown mucus plugs.

What is an aspergilloma?

A ball of fungus and debris that forms in a preexisting cavity. Can form in bronchiectatic airways in a cystic fibrosis adolescent. Symptomatic when eroding into nearby arteries

What is invasive pulmonary aspergillosis?

Deadly form of *Aspergillus* that happens in immunocompromised patients. Symptoms are insidious in onset over days to months. Symptoms can be fever, dry cough, dyspnea, pleuritic chest pain and mild hemoptysis, and life-threatening pulmonary hemorrhage.

Where does disseminated aspergillosis in immunocompromised patients likely to go?

Endophthalmitis, endocarditis, various organ abscesses

What is the treatment of choice for *Aspergillus* infection? For aspergilloma?

Voriconazole with or without caspofungin (textbooks often state: amphotericin B with flucytosine). Treatment for aspergilloma is resection.

What fungus is found in the Ohio and Mississippi river valleys, grows in soil contaminated by bird droppings, and causes pneumonia with intense exposure?

Histoplasma capsulatum

What type of spores does *Histoplasma* form?

Dimorphic fungus that forms microconidia

What type of cell wall does *Histoplasma* have?

Thin cell wall with no capsule

What type of cells does *H. capsulatum* infect and what is expected on lung tissue biopsy?

Cells of the reticuloendothelial system (e.g., macrophages). Oval yeast cells within macrophages are seen microscopically. Can cause hepatosplenomegaly

What dimorphic fungus is endemic to the eastern United States, and rarely in Latin America, and commonly causes pneumonia, although dissemination may result in ulcerated granulomas of other sites?

Blastomyces dermatitidis

How is *B. dermatitidis* diagnosed?

Tissue biopsy demonstrating thick-walled yeast cells with single broad-based buds

How is *Blastomyces* transmitted?

Inhaled conidia (budding spores). Common on rotting wood in the eastern United States

Which systemic mycosis causes *valley fever* in the San Joaquin Valley of California?

Coccidioides immitis

What are characteristic gross and microscopic pathology findings in lung tissue samples from patients infected with *Coccidioides*?

Gross pathology showing caseating granulomas with or without necrosis and cavitation and calcified pulmonary lesions. Microscopic examination of tissue specimens stained with silver revealing spherules filled with endospores

How is *Coccidioides* transmitted?

Inhalation of arthrospores (jointed spores) into the lungs

What are the three important sites of disseminated disease for *Coccidioides*?	1. Meninges 2. Bone 3. Skin
What opportunistic fungus is found in soil containing bird (especially pigeon) droppings and causes lung infection that is often asymptomatic or may produce pneumonia, especially in the immunocompromised patients?	*Cryptococcus neoformans*
Describe the preparation and characteristic appearance of *C. neoformans* under microscope: What sensitive test is used to diagnose *C. neoformans*?	India ink preparation shows budding yeasts surrounded by a wide, unstained capsule that is surrounded by a dark background. Latex agglutination test for polysaccharide capsular antigen
What is a major cause of pneumonia in HIV patients and is an AIDS-defining organism?	*Pneumocystis jiroveci* (formerly *Pneumocystis carinii*). Most infections are dormant until immunosuppressed, as in AIDS.
Describe the clinical picture of *Pneumocystis* pneumonia (PCP):	Diffuse, interstitial pneumonia
What is the characteristic appearance of a CXR for PCP?	Diffuse, patchy, "ground glass," bilateral appearance
What kind of microbiological testing is done to identify PCP?	Methenamine silver stain or DFA (direct fluorescence antigen) test of induced expectorant or bronchoalveolar lavage
How does PCP affect the lung walls?	*Pneumocystis jiroveci* damages type I pneumocytes causing increased permeability and foamy, honeycomb appearance.
What is the primary treatment and prophylaxis for PCP?	Trimethoprim and sulfamethoxazole Bactrim), or pentamidine/dapsone. Start when CD4 is less than 200 cell/mL.

Table 47.1 Table of Common Associations for Pneumonia

Keyword	Likely Diagnosis
Alcoholic	*Klebsiella, S. pneumoniae*
Elderly in nursing home facility	Gram-negative rods
Prisoners, immigrants	TB
Atypical pneumonia in patient from California or bordering areas	Coccidioidomycosis (valley fever), Hantavirus
Cystic fibrosis, bronchiectasis	*Pseudomonas aeruginosa*
Pneumonia symptoms with diarrhea or recent attendance at conference	*Legionella*
Immunosuppressed with large amounts of hemoptysis	Aspergillosis
HIV	*Pneumocystis jiroveci (P. carinii)* or TB
Exposure to bats, spelunking	*Histoplasma capsulatum*
Exposure to birds	*Chlamydia psittaci*
Exposure to rabbits	*Francisella tularensis*
Lung abscess	*Staphylococcus aureus*, oral anaerobes, TB, fungi
COPD/smoking	*Haemophilus influenzae, P. aeruginosa, Legionella, S. pneumoniae, M. catarrhalis*

CHAPTER 48

Gastrointestinal System

What are the four primary enteric host defenses against pathogens?	1. Gastric acid 2. Intestinal motility 3. Normal enteric flora (crowds out pathogenic species) 4. Intestinal immunity (immunoglobulins and Peyer's patches)
Through what route are almost all gastrointestinal (GI) pathogens taken in?	Oral route. However, keep in mind that many diseases that do not have predominant GI symptoms can also be acquired via the fecal-oral route (e.g., polio and botulism).

BACTERIAL GASTRITIS AND ULCERS

What species of bacteria is strongly urease-positive and causes pathology in the stomach?	*Helicobacter pylori*
Why is urease important to *H. pylori*?	Urease converts urea to ammonium ion (and CO_2) which neutralizes the stomach pH allowing the bacteria to survive.
What diseases are associated with *H. pylori* infection?	Gastritis and peptic ulcers
Where does *H. pylori* cause ulcers?	In the gastric antrum and the duodenum
Pathology Correlate: What are the four histologic zones of a chronic ulcer (superficial to deep)?	1. Necrotic tissue 2. Inflammation 3. Granulation tissue 4. Scar tissue at the base
For what cancers *is Helicobacter pylori* infection a risk factor?	Gastric carcinoma and mucosal-associated lymphoid tissue (MALT) lymphomas

What three methods can be used to diagnose *H. pylori* infection?	1. Serology antibody test 2. *Urea breath* test in which the radiolabeled CO_2 given off by radiolabeled urea is detected 3. Culture of biopsy from endoscopy
What is the combination of medications used to treat *H. pylori* infection?	The original treatment regimen includes the triple therapy of bismuth salts, metronidazole, and either ampicillin or tetracycline. The current regimen of choice is a proton pump inhibitor, amoxicillin, and clarithromycin (available as Prevpac).
What are the three curved gram-negative rods that cause disease in the GI tract?	1. *Helicobacter pylori* 2. *Campylobacter jejuni* 3. *Vibrio* species

TOXIGENIC BACTERIAL DIARRHEA

Which two species of bacteria are the main culprits for diarrhea caused by preformed toxins?	1. *Staphylococcus aureus* 2. *Bacillus cereus*
Which five bacteria are the main culprits for bacterial diarrhea caused by toxin production in vivo?	1. Clostridium perfringens 2. *Clostridium difficile* 3. *Bacillus cereus* (produces toxins both in vivo and preformed) 4. Enterotoxigenic *Escherichia coli* (ETEC) 5. *Vibrio cholerae*
What are the stool findings for diarrhea caused by toxigenic bacteria?	Generally unremarkable, no white blood cells (WBCs) or red blood cells (RBCs) (except *C. difficile*, stool may contain cytotoxin)
What are the signs and symptoms of diarrhea caused by preformed bacterial toxins?	Early-onset diarrhea (<6 hours), more vomiting than diarrhea, illness of short duration (<12 hours), and no fever
What are the signs and symptoms of diarrhea caused by bacterial toxin production in vivo?	Later-onset (12–24 hours), abdominal cramping, watery diarrhea. With the exception of *E. coli*, the symptoms typically resolve within 24 hours; *E. coli* symptoms last up to 5 days.

Which gram-positive coccus causes watery diarrhea via a superantigen enterotoxin that is acid-stable?

Staphylococcus aureus (symptom of vomiting is usually more prominent than diarrhea). Note that since the bacterium is acid-stable, it is not deactivated by gastric acid.

Can the *S. aureus* toxin be deactivated by boiling?

Yes, but the toxin is fairly resistant to heat so boiling must take place greater than 10 minutes at 60°C.

Which gram-positive rod causes diarrhea via two enterotoxins, one that is heat-stable and one that resembles cholera toxin?

Bacillus cereus

What is the mechanism of action for the two toxins of *B. cereus*?

The toxin adenosine diphosphate (ADP)-ribosylates a G protein, stimulating adenylate cyclase and resulting in an increased cyclic adenosine monophosphate (cAMP) level in the enterocyte. The other toxin is a superantigen similar to *S. aureus* in action.

Of the two enterotoxins produced by *B. cereus*, which one is produced in vivo and which one is preformed?

The cholera-like toxin is produced in vivo while the superantigen enterotoxin is preformed.

Why does *B. cereus* survive boiling of food while *S. aureus* does not?

Bacillus cereus produces heat-resistant spores; *S. aureus* does not produce spores.

What organism produces a watery diarrhea with classic findings of rice-water stool and a remarkable amount of fluid loss (7–8 L/d)?

Vibrio cholerae

What two things must occur in order for *V. cholerae* to cause disease?

1. The bacteria must colonize the small intestine.
2. Bacteria must secrete enterotoxin.

Does *V. cholerae* have a high or low ID50?

High. *Vibrio cholerae* is sensitive to gastric acid so approximately 10^6 organisms are required for the bacteria to colonize the small intestine, unless the patient is on antacids.

What is the reservoir for *V. cholerae* infection?

Contaminated water and food from contaminated water (e.g., seafood)

Is *V. cholerae* gram-positive or gram-negative? Is it a rod, coccus, or spirochete?	Gram-negative rod but it looks comma shaped. So do not be fooled, it is not a spirochete.
What do the two subunits, A (active) and B (binding), in the cholera enterotoxin do?	The B subunit binds to a ganglioside receptor on the enterocyte. After binding of the B subunit, the A subunit can then be inserted into the cytosol where it irreversibly activates glomerulosclerosis (Gs) protein through ADP-ribosylation.
What happens after cholera toxin activates Gs protein?	The active Gs protein causes increased stimulation of membrane-bound adenylate cyclase, which in turn results in increased production of cAMP. cAMP then leads to active secretion of chloride and inhibits absorption of sodium. This creates an osmotic force, resulting in a massive loss of water into the intestinal lumen.
What does the CTXφ virus have to do with *V. cholerae*?	The CTXφ virus is a bacteriophage that encodes the cholera enterotoxin. Cholera acquires the toxin through lysogenic conversion.
What are the signs and symptoms associated with cholera?	Because of massive volume loss and electrolyte abnormalities, patients exhibit hypotension, acidosis (from losing HCO_3^-), hypokalemia, hyponatremia, and possibly a dilutional hypernatremia from fluid loss. Acute tubular necrosis can eventually ensue and lead to death. Mortality is 40% untreated.
What is the treatment for cholera?	Intravenous (IV) or oral fluid replacement is imperative as rate of fluid loss is almost as dramatic as exsanguination. Antibiotics are not necessary, but tetracycline or quinolones can reduce the duration of diarrhea.
What preventive measures exist against cholera?	Public health measures are important (e.g., sanitation); vaccination is only 50% effective for 3 to 6 months and it does not prevent transmission; antibiotics are not effective in preventing epidemics.
Do patients acquire immunity to cholera after infection?	Yes. Prior infection induces a secretory immunoglobulin A (IgA) antibody.

What is the most common cause of diarrhea in hospitalized patients?

Clostridium difficile

What is the classic finding on the colonic mucosa associated with diarrhea caused by *C. difficile*?

Pseudomembranes, hence the disease is called pseudomembranous colitis

Considering that *C. difficile* is carried in the GI tract of 3% of normal people, what is the usual underlying cause of diarrhea?

Antibiotics kill the natural flora of the gut allowing an overgrowth of *C. difficile*. However, *C. difficile* is mainly a nosocomial infection.

What antibiotic is classically associated with pseudomembranous colitis?

Clindamycin is classically associated with pseudomembranous colitis.

What is the most common antibiotic that causes pseudomembranous colitis?

Cephalosporins are the most common cause of *C. difficile* pseudomembranous colitis because they are used much more frequently than clindamycin.

What is the treatment for pseudomembranous colitis?

Stop the offending antibiotic causing diarrhea and treat the *C. difficile* infection with oral vancomycin. Oral metronidazole is no longer considered first-line treatment but is still classically a treatment choice on board examinations.

What species of bacteria causes both gas gangrene and food poisoning?

Clostridium perfringens

What is the mechanism of action of the *C. perfringens* enterotoxin?

It is a superantigen similar to staphylococcal enterotoxin.

What protective characteristic of the bacteria makes them heat resistant?

Clostridium perfringens produces heat-resistant spores.

What is the laboratory diagnosis for diarrhea caused by *C. perfringens*?

There is none. Be careful not to confuse this with gas gangrene which is caused by the same bacteria. In the case of gas gangrene, tissue samples can be cultured on blood agar to yield double zone hemolysis or they can be cultured on egg yolk agar to show clearing. Stool cultures do not show *C. perfringens* diarrheal infection.

Which gram-negative rod is the principal cause of diarrheal illness in travelers and exists in more than 1000 different antigenic strains?

Enterotoxigenic *E. coli* (ETEC)

What two virulence factors must be present in order for ETEC to cause disease?	1. Pili (allow attachment of bacteria to mucosal surfaces in jejunum and ileum) 2. Enterotoxins If only one of these virulence factors is present, then the bacteria will not cause disease.
What are the two main types of toxins produced by ETEC and what are their mechanisms of action?	1. Heat-labile toxin (LT), which acts through a mechanism similar to cholera toxin (activates adenylate cyclase) 2. Heat-stable toxin (ST), which causes diarrhea by activating guanylate cyclase
What type of agar is *E. coli* grown on?	MacConkey agar yielding pink colonies (lactose fermenting). Note that not all *E. coli* are lactose fermenting (e.g., genetic recombination often uses *E. coli* that cannot ferment lactose).
What is the treatment for ETEC-associated diarrhea?	As with most watery diarrheas, fluid replacement is most important, but antibiotics shorten the duration of illness (typically fluoroquinolones or trimethoprim-sulfamethoxazole [TMP-SMX]).

INVASIVE BACTERIAL DIARRHEA

What is the classic symptom of diarrhea caused by organisms that invade the enteric mucosa?	Bloody diarrhea
What are the four main bacterial causes of bloody diarrhea?	1. *Shigella* 2. *Salmonella* 3. *Campylobacter* 4. *Escherichia coli* O157:H7
Of the four major causes of invasive diarrhea, which two do not ferment lactose?	1. *Shigella* 2. *Salmonella*
What are some other bacteria that can cause a bloody diarrhea?	*Yersinia enterocolitica*, *Vibrio parahaemolyticus*, enteroinvasive *E. coli* (EIEC), *C. difficile*, *Bacillus anthracis* (rare)

What does methylene blue staining indicate?

Leukocytes are present in the stool. This indicates an invasive organism (*Shigella, Salmonella, Campylobacter, E. coli* O157:H7) and not one of the toxin-producing organisms (except *C. difficile*).

Which curved gram-negative rod causes a bloody diarrhea and is associated with Guillain-Barré syndrome?

Campylobacter jejuni

Which is the most common cause of diarrhea worldwide: *Shigella*, *Salmonella*, or *Campylobacter*?

Campylobacter

What is the reservoir for *C. jejuni*?

Domestic animals such as dogs, cattle, and chickens

What is the clinical course of the disease?

Usually causes enterocolitis with initial watery stools, then lower abdominal pain, bloody mucopurulent diarrhea, and fever. Symptoms usually resolve in 7 days.

What autoimmune diseases can develop subsequent to GI infection with *Campylobacter*?

Guillain-Barré syndrome, reactive arthritis

How is a laboratory diagnosis made?

Campylobacter jejuni must be grown under special conditions to select it. Namely, a blood agar and antibiotic coupled with a temperature of 42°C and an atmosphere of 10% CO_2 and 5% O_2.

What is the treatment for *C. jejuni* diarrhea?

Ciprofloxacin or erythromycin can both be given to shorten the duration of symptoms and to prevent the spread of disease to others.

Does *Shigella* have a high or low ID50?

Very low. Just hundred organisms can cause disease.

What is the animal reservoir for *Shigella*?

None, it only infects humans.

Does *Shigella* cause disease through toxin production or enteroinvasion of the mucosa?

Through invasion of the mucosa. Mutated strains without the Shiga toxin still cause disease, but mutated strains that cannot invade do not cause disease.

What is the clinical course of the disease?	Incubation period of 1 to 3 days, followed by abdominal cramping, fevers, and watery diarrhea for the next 1 to 2 days. Then bloody mucus stools of low volume with rectal urgency and tenesmus with symptoms resolving after a week
Does everyone with shigellosis get grossly bloody diarrhea?	No, only 40% get gross blood; patients with *Shigella dysenteriae* are more likely to have severe disease than patient with *Shigella sonnei* or other *Shigella* species.
What is the treatment for shigellosis?	For mild disease, antibiotics are given more to prevent the spread of the bug than to treat the disease. For severe cases, fluoroquinolones or TMP-SMX is given. As always with diarrhea, fluid replacement is essential.
Which species of bacteria that produces a bloody diarrhea can be distinguished from *Shigella* by their ability to produce H_2S?	*Salmonella*
Is the ID50 for *Salmonella* higher or lower than *Shigella*?	Much higher. Approximately 100,000 organisms are required. The organism is susceptible to gastric acid, so patients on antacid and/or with a gastrectomy are more susceptible to infection.
What are the three clinical syndromes that *Salmonella* can cause?	1. *Salmonella* enterocolitis 2. *Salmonella* bacteremia 3. Typhoid fever (do not confuse typhoid fever with typhus) Note that while *Salmonella* enterocolitis is the only syndrome that affects the GI system primarily, the intestine is the portal of entry in all three cases.
What is the mode of transmission for *Salmonella*?	Domestic pets, poultry, and human beings. *Salmonella typhi* is only transmitted by human beings.
What is the clinical course of *Salmonella* enterocolitis?	Fever, abdominal cramps, bloody or watery diarrhea. Eighty percent of patients will have fecal leukocytes. Symptoms usually resolve within 7 days, though stool cultures can be positive for more than 2 months in 5% to 10% of patients.

What is the treatment for *Salmonella* enterocolitis?

Primarily fluid and electrolyte replacement. Antibiotics should generally be avoided as they do not reduce symptoms or duration of disease and may even prolong excretion of organisms and encourage carrier state. So ciprofloxacin, chloramphenicol, ampicillin, and TMP-SMX are given only to neonates, patients with chronic disease, atherosclerosis, or immunocompromised.

What organism in particular causes typhoid fever?

Salmonella typhi

At what histologic site does *S. typhi* replicate during intestinal invasion?

Within the macrophages concentrated at Peyer's patches. This causes hypertrophy and eventual necrosis leading to severe abdominal pain and subsequent ileal perforation.

What is the pathogenesis of typhoid fever during primary bacteremia?

After 5 to 7 days of replication in the Peyer's patches, the *S. typhi* seeds into the reticuloendothelial system (liver, bone marrow, spleen) through the lymphatic system and blood stream. They continue to undergo intracellular replication.

What happens during secondary bacteremia?

Salmonella typhi returns to the bowel through roundabout means. After 3 to 5 days of primary bacteremia, infection is established in the gallbladder where the chronic carrier state can persist. *Salmonella typhi* can silently shed from the biliary tract into the intestine (e.g., Typhoid Mary).

What are the symptoms during the stage of intestinal invasion?

Few symptoms. Mild abdominal pain and sometimes constipation or diarrhea

What are the symptoms during primary bacteremia?

Fever and *rose spots* on skin of abdomen. Once seeding takes hold in the reticuloendothelial system (RES), patients have hepatosplenomegaly.

What are rose spots?

Erythematous macular skin lesions characteristic of *S. typhi* infections

What are the signs and symptoms during secondary bacteremia?

Fever/pulse dissociation (high fever with a slow pulse), leukopenia, thrombocytopenia, slightly elevated liver function tests (LFTs)

What are the symptoms in chronic carriers?	Usually none, but these patients are a public health concern as they are reservoirs for infection.
At what stages is the blood culture positive and at what stages is the stool culture positive?	Blood cultures are positive during secondary bacteremia. The stool culture can be transiently positive during intestinal invasion but is always positive in chronic carriers.
What is the treatment for acute typhoid fever?	Fluoroquinolones or third-generation cephalosporin or azithromycin in patients with acute disease
What is the treatment for chronic carriers?	Long-term (6 weeks) high-dose ciprofloxacin works 80% of the time in patients without gallstones but only 25% of the time in patients with gallstones. Patients who fail therapy require a cholecystectomy.
Which gram-negative rod has strains of bacteria that can produce both a watery diarrhea and a bloody diarrhea? The bloody diarrhea variant is the bane of fast food beef.	*Escherichia coli*
What specific *E. coli* strain produces enterohemorrhagic diarrhea?	*Escherichia coli* O157:H7 (EHEC)
Why does *E. coli* O157:H7 produce bloody diarrhea while other strains of *E. coli* do not?	Probably because the O157:H7 strain has a verotoxin that kills cells of the gut mucosa
How does *E. coli* O157:H7 acquire the verotoxin?	Through lysogenic conversion
In laboratory diagnosis, how is *E. coli* O157:H7 distinguished from other *E. coli* strains?	It does not ferment sorbitol.
Should antibiotics be used in the treatment of diarrhea caused by *E. coli* O157:H7?	No. Treating with antibiotics predisposes to hemolytic-uremic syndrome (HUS) which is potentially life threatening.
What is HUS?	Acute kidney failure, hemolytic anemia, microvascular coagulation, and thrombocytopenia

What other organism is known to cause hemorrhagic diarrhea and HUS?

Shigella, although 70% of hemorrhagic diarrhea-associated HUS in the United States is caused by EHEC.

Other than *C. jejuni*, what curved gram-negative rod causes a bloody diarrhea?

Vibrio parahaemolyticus

What is the source for *V. parahaemolyticus*?

Contaminated seafood

What species of bacteria causes fever, diarrhea, and abdominal pain and is commonly confused with appendicitis?

Yersinia enterocolitica

VIRAL DIARRHEA

What are the typical histologic findings in a patient with viral gastroenteritis?

Mild mononuclear infiltration with blunting of intestinal villi

What is the pathogenesis of viral diarrhea?

A clear pathogenic mechanism is unknown, although viruses directly damage the small intestinal villi and may interfere with absorption and enzymatic activity. Rotavirus produces an enterotoxin that may contribute to diarrhea.

What is the route of transmission for viral gastroenteritis?

Fecal-oral transmission

What are the typical signs and symptoms?

Low-to-moderate grade fevers, nausea, vomiting, abdominal cramps, and diarrhea. No WBCs or blood in stool

What is the course of this disease in healthy adults?

Mild and self-limited

Is diarrhea a serious medical condition for children?

In the United States, approximately 400 children die from complications of diarrhea each year. However, it is estimated that 2 million children worldwide die from complications of diarrhea each year. Children are more susceptible to secondary dehydration and secondary nutrient malabsorption.

What two virus families are responsible for the majority of viral gastroenteritis?

1. Norwalk virus (also known as norovirus)
2. Rotavirus

Which of the above virus families targets adults and which targets infants/young children?

Rotavirus targets infants and young children while Norwalk virus targets adults.

Which virus is associated with outbreaks in group settings, such as cruise ships, camps, and dorms?

Norwalk virus

What makes Norwalk virus in particular infectious?

Low infectious dose, virus excreted in stool for several weeks after recovery, and resistance to inactivation by chlorination and desiccation (so be more wary about where you swim)

What is the treatment for diarrhea caused by Norwalk and/or rotavirus?

No antiviral treatments exist. Treatment is supportive and aims at maintaining hydration.

What preventive measures can be taken to avoid viral diarrhea outbreaks?

Public health measures, such as sewage disposal, and personal hygiene are likely to prevent infection.

Which virus causes a nonbloody diarrhea primarily in children younger than the age of 2 years?

Adenovirus

PROTOZOAL DIARRHEA

Which two protozoa produce nonbloody diarrhea?

1. *Giardia lamblia*
2. *Cryptosporidium parvum*

Which bug causes amebic dysentery (bloody diarrhea)?

Entamoeba histolytica

What is more effective in killing *E. histolytica*, boiling or chlorination?

Boiling. They are heat susceptible but chlorination does not kill them, so beware of the public pool.

How is amebic dysentery spread?

Fecal-oral route. Ingestion of cysts in contaminated food or water

What group in America has a higher incidence of amebic dysentery?

Homosexual males

Pathology Correlate: What finding on histology is associated with amebic dysentery?

Flask-shaped ulcers form once the ameba invades colonic glands and reaches the submucosa.

How is the aspirated substance from *E. histolytica* liver abscesses classically described?	Brownish-yellow pus that looks like anchovy paste
What distinguishes *E. histolytica* from other amebae?	A cyst with four nuclei
What is the treatment for *E. histolytica* infection?	Metronidazole
How is *G. lamblia* spread?	Fecal-oral or anal-oral route
What groups in America have a higher incidence of giardiasis?	Homosexual males and hikers who drink from freshwater sources
Is *Giardia* common in the United States?	Yes, approximately 5% of stool samples in America contain *Giardia* cysts.
Which site of the GI tract does *G. lamblia* primarily infect?	Duodenum
What are the symptoms associated with giardiasis?	Nonbloody, foul-smelling diarrhea, flatulence, and weight loss with chronic disease. No fever
How is giardiasis diagnosed?	Trophozoites in stool have a characteristic appearance, pear-shaped with two nuclei, four pairs of flagella, and a suction disk. Sometimes small intestine aspirate (string test) or biopsy is needed.
What is the treatment for giardiasis?	Metronidazole
For what population of patients in particular is cryptosporidiosis a major concern?	Immunocompromised patients, especially AIDS patients

OTHER GI INFECTIONS

Which virus, and to which family of viruses does it belong to, causes worldwide food-related acute hepatitis?	Hepatitis A virus (HAV), picornavirus
Which virus, and to which family of viruses does it belong to, causes contaminated water-associated acute hepatitis noted for its high mortality in pregnant women in the developing countries?	Hepatitis E virus (HEV). HEV is now classified into its own hepevirus genus with no assigned family.

Which virus, and to which family of viruses does it belong to, causes acute hepatitis acquired through contaminated needles that develops into chronic hepatitis 85% to 90% of the time?

Hepatitis C virus (HCV), flavivirus

Which virus, and to which family of viruses does it belong to, causes acute or chronic hepatitis depending on the method of transmission?

Hepatitis B virus (HBV), hepadnavirus; vertical (neonatal) transmission associated with a high risk of chronic hepatitis, horizontal (needle/transfusion) transmission associated with acute hepatitis, and a much lower risk of chronic hepatitis

Which virus, and to which family of viruses does it belong to, causes fulminant hepatitis and is a defective virus?

Hepatitis D virus (HDV), delta virus; HDV requires HBV coinfection

Which hepatitis viruses are enveloped? Which are transmitted through fecal-oral route?

HBV, HCV, and HDV are enveloped viruses and cannot survive the GI tract. HAV and HEV are nonenveloped and transmitted via the fecal-oral route.

Chronic infection with what parasite can cause portal hypertension (most common cause worldwide), cirrhosis, and even pulmonary hypertension?

Schistosoma mansoni

What two species of parasites can potentially cause intestinal obstruction causing patients to present with acute abdominal pain?

1. *Ascaris lumbricoides*
2. *Diphyllobothrium latum*

What type of anemia is *D. latum* infection associated with? Why?

Megaloblastic anemia. Diphyllobothriumlatum may interfere with vitamin B_{12} adsorption.

What two species of nematodes can cause microcytic anemia?

1. *Ancylostoma duodenale* (hookworm)
2. *Necator americanus* (hookworm)

What nematode is a common cause of perianal pruritus in young children?

Enterobius vermicularis

What cestodes cause tapeworm infections?

Taenia solium (pork), *Taenia saginata* (beef), *D. latum* (fish), *Echinococcus granulosus* (dog).

CHAPTER 49

Genitourinary System

URINARY TRACT INFECTIONS

What types of infections are considered urinary tract infections (UTIs)?

Lower tract infection (e.g., acute cystitis, bladder) or upper tract infection (e.g., acute pyelonephritis, kidney)

What is the major mode of bacterial entry in the genitourinary tract?

Ascending periurethral infection. Hematogenous spread is also seen in immunocompromised patients and neonates.

What are the common symptoms of uncomplicated acute cystitis?

Dysuria, increased urinary urgency, and suprapubic pain

What is the most common cause of uncomplicated acute cystitis?

Escherichia coli causes 80% to 85% of all uncomplicated acute cystitis.

Which family of bacteria that causes UTIs is known for reducing nitrates to nitrites?

Enterobacteriaceae, which includes the bacteria *E. coli*, causes nitrites to appear in urine analysis.

What is an important cause of uncomplicated acute cystitis in newly sexually active females?

Staphylococcus saprophyticus, although *E. coli* is still more common

Why are females more susceptible to UTIs than males?

Females have a shorter urethra, which is in close proximity to the rectum. This allows for the increased incidence of UTIs.

Why are certain females more susceptible to recurrent UTIs?

A subset of females experience recurrent UTIs due to increased mucosal receptivity to bacteria adhesion

What is the treatment of choice for uncomplicated acute cystitis?

Three-day treatment with trimethoprim-sulfamethoxazole (TMP-SMX) or fluoroquinolones. Single-dose therapy sterilizes the urine but allows recrudescent infection from periurethral tissue.

What are complicated UTIs?

Complicated UTIs are associated with upper tract infection, diabetes, male sex, pregnancy, hospital- or catheter-related infections, and anatomical/surgical variants. Bacterial resistance is more common and requires prolonged treatment with broad-spectrum antibiotics. Uncomplicated UTIs are limited to simple cystitis in healthy women.

Why does a UTI in a male warrant further workup, including imaging studies of the urinary tract?

In males, UTIs (especially recurrent UTIs) are frequently associated with an anatomical abnormalities such as urinary obstruction due to benign prostatic hyperplasia and urethral stricture.

What common cause of UTIs is known to have swarming motility?

Proteus mirabilis

What bacteria are associated with struvite (staghorn renal calculi)?

Ureaplasma urealyticum, P. mirabilis, Corynebacterium urealyticum, Pseudomonas, Klebsiella, Staphylococcus, and *Mycoplasma*

What enzyme allows them to form struvite stones?

Urease which cleaves urea forming ammonia, which raises the pH leading to precipitation of phosphate, carbonate, and magnesium

What are common causes of catheter-related acute cystitis?

Escherichia coli, Serratia marcescens, Enterobacter cloacae, Klebsiella pneumonia, P. mirabilis, and *Pseudomonas aeruginosa*

What is the treatment of choice for complicated acute cystitis?

Minimum 7 to 14 days treatment with fluoroquinolones

What are common symptoms and findings of upper tract infection?

Fevers, chills, flank pain, and costovertebral angle (CVA) tenderness. Additionally, the presence of white cell casts on urinalysis supports a diagnosis of pyelonephritis. Sometimes these features are absent and upper tract infection is diagnosed after failure of short-course therapy for apparent lower tract infection.

What is the most common cause of acute pyelonephritis?

Escherichia coli, in more than 70% cases (second most common *S. saprophyticus*)

Pathology Correlate: What is the gross pathologic appearance of pyelonephritis?

Focal, pale, raised abscesses on the cortical surface

What is an important virulence factor for *E. coli* that enables it to cause acute cystitis and acute pyelonephritis?	P-pili, which help *E. coli* bind to uroepithelial cells. Almost all *E. coli* which cause acute pyelonephritis have P-pili.
How is acute pyelonephritis treated?	Commonly with oral fluoroquinolones or parental ceftriaxone for 14 days. However, therapy should be based on results of urine culture with sensitivities.
What are the signs and symptoms of acute prostatitis?	Fever, chills, malaise, obstructive symptoms, dysuria
What are the common causes of acute prostatitis?	Same organisms that cause acute cystitis, mainly *E. coli* and *Proteus*
How is acute prostatitis treated?	Patients require long-term (weeks) therapy that should be organism directed. If possible, TMP-SMX or quinolones should be used because of better penetration into the prostate.
How does chronic prostatitis present?	Many are asymptomatic or have signs of a lower UTI.
How is chronic prostatitis treated?	Minimum 6 weeks of fluoroquinolones (ideally guided by sensitivities from urine or semen culture)
Pathology Correlate: What form of prostatitis is characterized by multinucleated giant cells?	Granulomatous prostatitis, caused by disseminated tuberculosis and fungal infections.

VAGINAL INFECTIONS

What species of bacteria helps maintain a normal vaginal pH of 3.8 to 4.5?	*Lactobacillus*
What species of protozoa causes a foul-smelling vaginal discharge with itching and burning and on physical examination shows a fiery red cervix?	*Trichomonas vaginalis*
Describe the morphology of *T. vaginalis*:	Pear-shaped organism with four anterior flagella and corkscrew motility
What is the treatment of choice for *T. vaginalis* infection?	Metronidazole

Pharmacology Correlate: What is the mechanism of action for metronidazole and what types of organisms is it effective against?

Metronidazole is reduced by the electron transport chain in anaerobic bacteria to active form and then it causes DNA-strand breakage and destabilization. It is effective against anaerobic bacteria and *Trichomonas* and *Entamoeba*; there is virtually no resistance.

What species of bacteria causes a yellow-greenish malodorous vaginal discharge with increased vaginal pH (> 5)?

Gardnerella vaginalis (as part of bacterial vaginosis, which is probably due to a mix of *Gardnerella* and anaerobes overgrowing the normal *Lactobacillus*)

How is bacterial vaginosis diagnosed?

Demonstration of clue cells on saline smear. Clue cells are vaginal squamous epithelial cells covered by bacteria cells.

What happens when 10% potassium hydroxide (KOH) is mixed with vaginal fluid from a patient with bacterial vaginosis?

The alkaline nature of 10% KOH releases volatile amines from the vaginal fluid leading to the characteristic fishy odor. Vaginal odor is the most common symptom; often the initial symptom and often occurs following sexual intercourse (semen is also alkaline).

What fungus causes a white cottage cheese-like vaginal discharge and shows pseudohyphae and budding yeast on microscopic examination?

Candida albicans

CHLAMYDIA

What is the most common cause of bacterial sexually transmitted disease (STD)? What structure does its cell wall lack?

Chlamydia trachomatis is the most common bacterial STD and is recognized by the fact that its cell wall lacks muramic acid.

***Chlamydia trachomatis* is also responsible for trachoma, the most common cause of preventable blindness in the world. What serotypes are especially known to cause blindness?**

Serotypes A, B, C are known to cause chronic infections and blindness especially in the African continent

Mnemonic: A = Africa, **B = B**lindness, **C = C**hronic infection

What diseases do serotypes D-K cause?	Types D-K cause urethritis, pelvic inflammatory disease, neonatal pneumonia, and neonatal conjunctivitis.
What disease do serotypes L1, L2, L3 cause?	Types L1, L2, and L3 are responsible for lymphogranuloma venereum, a disease that presents initially with a painless genital papule, which then proceeds to inguinal lymphadenopathy, and possibly genital elephantiasis **Mnemonic: L** serotype causes **L**ymphogranuloma venereum.
Pelvic inflammatory disease increases the risk of what complications?	Infertility and ectopic pregnancy
Why is *C. trachomatis* considered an obligate intracellular parasite?	*Chlamydia trachomatis* is unable to make its own ATP.
Which form of *C. trachomatis* is metabolically active, the reticulate body or elementary body?	The reticulate form is metabolically active, is found in cells, and replicates by fission. The elementary form is the infective form that enters cells by endocytosis. **Mnemonic: E** for entering. **R** for replicating.
What is Fitz-Hugh and Curtis syndrome?	An infection of the liver capsule secondary to pelvic inflammatory disease caused by *Neisseria gonorrhoeae* or *Chlamydia*. Patients present with right upper quadrant (RUQ) pain and sepsis.

GONORRHEA

What other bacterium is a common cause of pelvic inflammatory disease?	*Neisseria gonorrhoeae*
What are some morphologic and biochemical characteristics of *N. gonorrhoeae*?	*Neisseria gonorrhoeae* is described as gram-negative diplococci that ferment lactose but not maltose.
Gram-negative diplococci identified in which type of cell from a urethral swab is sufficient for diagnosis of *N. gonorrhoeae* infection?	Polymorphonuclear neutrophils (PMNs)

What is the ideal culture medium for *N. gonorrhoeae*?	Thayer-Martin [VCN] medium
What virulence factor of *N. gonorrhoeae* **makes it impossible for an effective vaccine to be produced?**	Pili, which allow it to attach to mucosal surfaces and inhibit phagocytic uptake. The pili have antigenic variation with more than one million variants, which hinders production of an effective vaccine.
What is the treatment of choice for *N. gonorrhoeae*?	Ceftriaxone (a third-generation cephalosporin). *Neisseria gonorrhoeae* are often resistant to penicillin due to β-lactamase production.

SYPHILIS

What species of bacteria causes a nontender ulcer that heals spontaneously after 2 to 6 weeks?	*Treponema pallidum*
Describe the stages of syphilis:	Primary syphilis presents with a painless chancre on the penis or labia and lasts 3 to 6 weeks. Secondary syphilis presents 1 to 3 months later after hematogenous spread of the organism and manifests as a skin rash that includes the palms and soles, as well as condyloma lata, a flat wart-like lesion in intertriginous regions (e.g., near the anus). Tertiary syphilis occurs years later in approximately 30% of untreated patients and can present with aortitis, tabes dorsalis, and gummas.
How is syphilis diagnosed?	Venereal Disease Research Laboratory (VDRL) (nonspecific), rapid plasma reagin (RPR) (nonspecific), and fluorescent treponemal antibody absorbed (FTA-ABS) (specific)
Which test remains positive for life after infection?	FTA-ABS
What type of staining/microscopy is needed to adequately visualize *T. pallidum*?	Dark-field microscopy is used to visualize the treponemas.

What is the treatment of choice for *T. pallidum* **infection?**	Penicillin G
What is the Jarisch-Herxheimer reaction?	A self-resolving reaction that occurs after antibiotic treatment for a spirochete disease and manifests as an increase in temperature, decrease in blood pressure, rigors and leukopenia, headache, chills, malaise; it results from the release of treponemal cell wall products after lysis by the antibiotics.
The likelihood of fetal infection during pregnancy can be decreased if the *T. pallidum* **infection is treated before what stage of gestation?**	*Treponema pallidum* infection does not seem to damage the fetus until after 20 weeks of gestation. **Mnemonic: TORCH** (**T**oxoplasmosis, **O**thers (syphilis), **R**ubella, **C**MV, **H**erpes/**H**IV)
Describe the ocular lesion commonly found in syphilis:	Argyll-Robertson pupil is caused by a midbrain lesion, leading to a pupil that constricts during accommodation, but not to light.

HSV

Which virus causes multiple recurrent painful vesicular lesions in the genital area?	Herpes simplex virus type 2 (HSV-2)
In which ganglia does HSV-2 commonly remain latent? HSV-1?	Typically HSV-2 remains latent in the sacral ganglia while HSV-1 remains latent in the trigeminal root ganglion.
What type of smear can be used to detect HSV infection? What are characteristic findings?	Tzanck smear (you would expect to see multinucleated giant cells). Tzanck smear has been largely replaced by immunofluorescent staining, which is able to distinguish between HSV-1, HSV-2, and varicella zoster virus (VZV).
Describe the structural and genetic characteristics of herpesvirus:	Enveloped icosahedral capsid with linear double-stranded DNA genome
Where does herpesvirus obtain its envelope?	Host nuclear membrane
Where is herpesvirus assembled?	Host nucleus

What is the treatment of choice for HSV infections? And what enzyme is required to activate the drug?

Acyclovir. Thymidine kinase

HPV

What is the most common STD in the United States?

Human papillomavirus (HPV). (*Chlamydia* is only the most common bacterial STD.)

HPV strains 16 and 18 are thought to cause cervical cancer by the inhibition of what tumor suppressor genes?

HPV 16 creates protein product E6, which inhibits p53; HPV 18 makes protein product E7, which inhibits the retinoblastoma (Rb) tumor suppressor gene.

Mnemonic: 16 is before **18, E6** is before **E7, p53 (P)** is before **Rb (R). 16 E6 p53/18 E7 Rb**

What strains of HPV cause anogenital warts (condyloma acuminatum)?

HPV strains 6 and 11

Pathology Correlate: what characteristic cytopathology would a Pap smear from a patient infected with HPV show?

Koilocytic cells or cells that show perinuclear cytoplasmic vacuolization with nuclear enlargement

OTHERS

What rare cancer is caused by *Schistosoma haematobium*?

Squamous cell carcinoma of the bladder usually in patients from Egypt. Most bladder cancers are transitional cell carcinomas.

What species of bacteria causes a painful genital lesion similar to the lesion seen in primary syphilis?

Haemophilus ducreyi
Mnemonic: *H. duCReYi causes patients to cry*

CHAPTER 50

Ears, Eyes, and Nervous System

EAR

What are the three most common causative microbes of acute otitis media?

1. *Streptococcus pneumoniae*
2. *Moraxella catarrhalis*
3. *Haemophilus influenza*

Mnemonic: **S**ick **M**essy **H**earing

What tests can be used to differentiate the most common causative *Streptococcus* species from other *Streptococcus* species?

Streptococcus pneumoniae is α-hemolytic and optochin-sensitive.

What is the antibiotic of choice in otitis media infections?

Amoxicillin is usually first-line treatment to cover *Moraxella*, *H. influenzae*, and *S. pneumoniae* empirically. However, penicillin-resistant *S. pneumoniae* is more common and amoxicillin-clavulanate (Augmentin) or a cephalosporin may be necessary.

What species of bacteria causes otitis externa characterized by pain with pulling of the outer ear and a recent history of swimming in a freshwater pond?

Pseudomonas aeruginosa (*Staphylococcus aureus* may also cause otitis externa but not associated with water source), although etiology commonly mixed bacteria

Malignant otitis media is a life-threatening *P. aeruginosa* infection generally found in patients with which comorbid condition?

Diabetes

EYES

Name the two most common organisms that cause sty (infection of the eyelids):	1. *Staphylococcus aureus* 2. *Propionibacterium acnes*
What are the primary symptoms associated with conjunctivitis?	Eyes "stuck shut" in the morning, erythema of the conjunctiva, and purulent (thick green/yellow = bacterial infection) or nonpurulent (watery = allergy/viral)
What bacteria are the most common causes of bacterial conjunctivitis by age group?	Neonates: *Neisseria gonorrhoeae, Chlamydia trachomatis, S. aureus* Infants and young children: *H. influenzae, Moraxella* Adults: *S. pneumoniae, S. aureus, C. trachomatis* Sexually active adults: *N. gonorrhoeae, C. trachomatis* (both very rare)
What three viruses are the most common cause of viral conjunctivitis?	1. Adenovirus (associated with iatrogenic outbreaks) 2. Coxsackievirus 3. Enterovirus 70
What is the leading cause of infectious blindness in the United States?	Herpes simplex virus 1 (HSV-1)
HSV-1 infects not just the conjunctiva, but also the cornea at the same time. What is it called when both the cornea and conjunctiva are inflamed?	Keratoconjunctivitis
What is the leading cause of preventable blindness in the world?	Ocular trachoma caused by *C. trachomatis* serotypes A, B, and C
How does infection with *C. trachomatis* cause blindness?	*Chlamydia trachomatis* causes the eyelids to evert onto the globe. The inturned eyelashes then rub against the cornea and cause severe scarring leading to blindness.
Which drugs can be used to prevent or treat ophthalmia neonatorum secondary to congenital *N. gonorrhoeae* infection and *C. trachomatis* infection?	Topical macrolide. Silver nitrate was historically used but discontinued due to complication of chemical conjunctivitis.

What organism is likely responsible for causing periorbital edema in a patient who recently traveled to South America?

Trypanosoma cruzi (Chagas disease)

By which two organisms are Chorioretinitis in neonates or AIDS patients are commonly caused?

1. *Toxoplasma* (neonates)
2. Cytomegalovirus (CMV) (AIDS patients)

What eye infection can congenital infection with rubella cause?

Cataract

What is the drug of choice for the treatment of ganciclovir-resistant CMV retinitis?

Foscarnet or cidofovir

MENINGITIS

What are some clinical signs and symptoms of meningitis?

Headache, photosensitivity, nuchal rigidity, and nausea/vomiting

What are the cerebrospinal fluid (CSF) findings for bacterial meningitis?

Elevated pressure, opaque CSF, increased white blood cells (WBCs) with predominantly polymorphonuclear neutrophils (PMNs), decreased glucose, and increased protein

What are the CSF findings for viral meningitis?

Normal to slightly elevated pressure, clear CSF, moderately elevated cells with predominantly lymphocytes, normal to slightly decreased glucose, normal to slightly increased protein

What three species of bacteria are the most common causes of neonatal meningitis?

Streptococcus agalactiae, Escherichia coli, and *Listeria monocytogenes*

What are some distinguishing biochemical characteristics of *S. agalactiae*?

Streptococcus agalactiae is part of normal oral and vaginal flora, hydrolyzes hippurate, has five serotypes, is bacitracin-resistant, has a sialic acid capsule, and is β-hemolytic.

What two species of bacteria are the most common causes of adult meningitis?

1. *Neisseria meningitidis*
2. *Streptococcus pneumoniae*

What was a major cause of childhood meningitis but number of cases has dramatically decreased since introduction of its vaccine?

Haemophilus influenzae

What species of bacteria is a leading cause of meningitis in neonates, pregnant women, and adults with renal transplants?

Listeria monocytogenes

What species of bacteria classically causes meningitis in new military recruits?

Neisseria meningitidis. It is also a frequent cause of meningitis in asplenic patients (cannot clear capsulated organisms) and patients deficient in complements C5-C8.

What is the treatment of choice for *N. meningitidis* meningitis? What is the prophylaxis of choice?

Third-generation cephalosporins (e.g., ceftriaxone) or penicillin. Prophylaxis with rifampin or ciprofloxacin

What diagnosis should be seriously considered in a patient with tuberculosis, nerve palsies, and low CSF glucose?

Tuberculous meningitis, while relatively uncommon in the United States, is common worldwide, and antibiotic treatment must be started immediately.

What are the most common viral causes of meningitis?

Enteroviruses (most common cause; poliovirus, echovirus, Coxsackievirus), human immunodeficiency virus (HIV), and HSV-2

What fungal organism is a leading cause of meningitis in AIDS patients?

Cryptococcus neoformans causes meningoencephalitis. Cryptococcal antigen in CSF should always be tested as well. The India ink test for encapsulated yeast is not commonly performed anymore.

ENCEPHALITIS

What are the common signs and symptoms of encephalitis?

Patients often also present with meningeal signs, but encephalitis usually presents with behavioral/personality changes, decreased level of consciousness, seizures, and confusion.

What are the most common causes of encephalitis?

Arboviruses (most common cause), HSV, and toxoplasma (in HIV patients)

Which families of viruses do Arboviruses, which are spread from either mosquito or tick species, include?

Flaviviruses (St. Louis encephalitis virus, West Nile virus), togaviruses (western and eastern equine encephalitis virus), bunyaviruses (California encephalitis virus), and reoviruses (Colorado tick fever virus)

What species of viruses are the leading causes of epidemic viral encephalitis in the United States?

West Nile virus (most common) and St. Louis encephalitis virus (second most common)

How often does encephalitis develop following West Nile virus infection?

Estimated only 1 in 150 infections results in meningitis or encephalitis.

How are birds involved in the spread and maintenance of West Nile virus?.

Birds typically develop sustained high levels of viremia but remain asymptomatic (although some species of birds also die from the disease). This helps spread and maintain a constant source of virus

What is the most important risk factor in predicting development of encephalitis, following infection with West Nile virus or St. Louis encephalitis virus?

Age. Elderly patients are significantly more likely to develop symptomatic infections.

What is the most common cause of fatal sporadic encephalitis in the United States?

HSV-1 encephalitis

Which HSV type causes encephalitis in neonates?

HSV-2

Pathology Correlate: Which lobes of the brain are usually affected by HSV encephalitis and what is seen histologically?

Hemorrhagic necrosis in the temporal and frontal lobes with Cowdry type A inclusions are pathognomonic of HSV encephalitis.

What are the most common parenchymal brain lesions in AIDS patients?

Toxoplasma encephalitis, HIV encephalopathy, primary central nervous system (CNS) lymphoma, and progressive multifocal leukoencephalopathy

What are the characteristic lesions in *Toxoplasma* encephalitis?

Multiple ring-enhancing lesions at the corticomedullary junction

Which virus, and to which family of viruses does it belong to, causes progressive multifocal leukoencephalopathy? How common is JC virus infection?

JC virus in the polyomavirus family. JC virus infections affect approximately 90% of general population but only reactivate with severe immunosuppression.

Pathology Correlate: What are the characteristic lesions of progressive multifocal leukoencephalopathy?

Multiple bilateral hypodense or hypointense lesions correspond to areas of demyelination in the cortical white matter as a result of JC virus infection of oligodendrocytes.

What species of protozoa causes meningoencephalitis in immunocompromised patients with dirty contact lenses?

Acanthamoeba

What species of protozoa causes an extremely deadly meningoencephalitis that typically follows swimming in freshwater during the summer? How does it enter the CNS?

Naegleria fowleri causes approximately 97% mortality rate in infected individuals, even young adults. It enters the CNS through the cribriform plate.

PRION

What is the main difference between normal and pathological prions?

Normal prions have α-helix formation while abnormal ones have β-pleated sheets.

Name five diseases that present as subacute spongiform encephalopathy:

1. Kuru
2. Creutzfeldt-Jakob
3. Gerstmann-Sträussler-Scheinker syndrome
4. Fatal familial insomnia
5. Scrapie

Pathology Correlate: What actually account for the "spongy" changes in these diseases?

Vacuoles within the gray matter

OTHER NEUROLOGICAL DISEASES

What virus causes lethargy, poor feeding, microcephaly, chorioretinitis, and periventricular calcifications in neonates?

CMV

What species of bacteria is associated with ascending paralysis?

Campylobacter jejuni (Guillain-Barré syndrome)

What species of bacteria causes Bell palsy? What species of viruses?

Borrelia burgdorferi; HSV-1, and less commonly varicella-zoster virus (VZV)

What virus causes motor paralysis and what type of neurons does it infect?

Polio virus and anterior horn motor neurons and sometimes West Nile virus

What neurological disease that presents with influenza-like symptoms with meningeal signs is caused by an arenavirus, typically from South America?

Lymphocytic choriomeningitis

What long-term neurological complication can arise from measles infection?

Subacute sclerosing panencephalitis, which develops 7 to 10 years after the initial measles virus infection and occurs typically in patients younger than 20 years

What increases the risk of developing subacute sclerosing panencephalitis?

Infection with the measles virus at an early age

What is the classic triad of congenital toxoplasmosis?

1. Chorioretinitis
2. Hydrocephalus
3. Intracranial calcifications

How is congenital toxoplasmosis acquired?

Classically with pregnant women handling cat litter boxes or eating undercooked lamb or beef

CHAPTER 51

Skin

BACTERIAL PATHOGENS

Name five species of bacteria that constitute normal flora of the skin:	1. *Staphylococcus aureus* (found in 20%–55% of people) 2. *Staphylococcus epidermidis* 3. *Propionibacterium acnes* 4. *Pseudomonas aeruginosa* 5. *Corynebacterium*
What common skin anaerobe is implicated in the pathogenesis of acne?	*Propionibacterium acnes*
What species of bacteria causes bullae and desquamated skin with epidermis that easily dislodges under pressure typically in children (Nikolsky sign)?	*Staphylococcus aureus* (scalded skin syndrome by epidermolytic toxin)
What other types of skin infections does S. *aureus* cause?	Folliculitis, furuncles, bullous impetigo, and wound infections
What is S. *aureus* toxic shock syndrome?	Systemic disease caused by superantigen toxic shock syndrome toxin 1 (TSST-1) that presents with fever, hypotension, multiorgan failure, and diffuse erythematous rash with desquamation on palms and soles
What is the mechanism of action of the TSST-1 toxin?	TSST-1 is a superantigen that stimulates release of large amounts of interleukin 1 (IL-1), IL-2, and tumor necrosis factor (TNF), leading to systemic shock.
How is S. *aureus* impetigo classically described and in what population is it most common?	Superficial skin infection with erythema, bullae, pustules, and a honey-colored crust that occurs usually on the face and extremities of children.

What other species of bacteria cause impetigo?

Streptococcus pyogenes

Why must *S. pyogenes* impetigo be treated?

Streptococcus pyogenes impetigo should be treated because of an association with poststreptococcal glomerulonephritis.

What disease is caused by *S. pyogenes* that presents with maculopapular rash classically described as a *sandpaper rash* and a *strawberry tongue*?

Scarlet fever cause by erythrogenic toxin

What is the mechanism of action of the erythrogenic toxin?

It acts as a superantigen; similar to the toxin produced by *S. aureus* in toxic shock syndrome.

Streptococcus pyogenes is also the leading cause of which superficial skin infection?

Cellulitis

Which inflammation-related enzyme produced by *S. pyogenes* is known as *spreading factor* because of its ability to enable the rapid spread of *S. pyogenes* in cellulitis?

Hyaluronidase, which degrades hyaluronic acid, is an important component of the subcutaneous tissue.

What are other important causes of cellulitis?

Staphylococcus aureus and occasionally gram-negative rods such as *Escherichia coli* and *Pasteurella multocida*

What two species of bacteria commonly cause intravenous catheter-related infections?

Staphylococcus epidermidis and *S. aureus*

What species of bacteria causes *rose spots*, which are rose-colored macules on the abdomen and is associated with high fever, constipation, a tender abdomen, and an enlarged spleen?

Salmonella typhi (typhoid fever)

What species of bacteria causes erythema migrans, an expanding, erythematous, nonpruritic rash with a clear center at the site of a tick bite?

Borrelia burgdorferi (Lyme disease)

What family of bacteria causes a rash characterized by petechiae and purpura following tick or louse bite?

Rickettsiae family, *Rickettsia rickettsii* (Rocky Mountain spotted fever), *Rickettsia typhi,* and *Rickettsia prowazekii* (typhus)

Which rickettsial disease causes an outward (centrifugal) spread of rash and which causes an inward (centripedal) spread?

The rash of typhus (*R. typhi* and *R. prowazekii*) begins on the trunk and spreads outward to the periphery. The rash of Rocky Mountain spotted fever (*R. rickettsii*) begins on the wrists and ankles, then spreads inward to the trunk and to the palms/soles.

What species of bacteria is the slowest-growing human bacterial pathogen, is cultured in mouse footpads or armadillos, and causes Hansen disease?

Mycobacterium leprae

Which form of leprosy involves a cell-mediated response that limits the growth of *M. leprae*, a positive lepromin skin test, and microscopic examination showing few acid-fast bacilli?

Tuberculoid leprosy

Pathology Correlate: What classic histology is tuberculoid leprosy associated with?

Granulomas containing giant cells

What are some clinical findings associated with tuberculoid leprosy?

A single or few skin lesions, which are hypopigmented, macular and anesthetic, and thickened superficial nerves that can be palpated; commonly ulnar, posterior tibial, and perineal

Which form of leprosy involves a poor cell-mediated response to *M. leprae*, a negative lepromin skin test, and microscopic examination showing a large number of acid-fast bacilli with foamy histiocytes?

Lepromatous leprosy

Describe the clinical findings associated with lepromatous leprosy:

Diffuse involvement of the skin with multiple nodular lesions, commonly resulting in the disfigurement of the hands and the face (termed leonine or lion-like facies). Involvement of the eyes, nerves, testes, and upper airway is also common.

What antibiotic is the mainstay of leprosy treatment, although use with additional drugs is now recommended because of emerging resistance?

Dapsone

What species of bacteria causes a black eschar with significant local edema that may progress to bacteremia and death if left untreated?

Bacillus anthrax, cutaneous anthrax acquired via implantation of spores into skin

What gram-positive anaerobe is a normal flora of the oral cavity but can cause oral/facial abscesses with *sulfur granules* draining through sinus tracts of the skin?

Actinomyces israelii (sulfur granules do not contain sulfur)

What species of bacteria causes a maculopapular rash on the palms and soles, moist lesions of the genitals, patchy alopecia, and constitutional symptoms?

Treponema pallidum (during secondary syphilis stage)

What is the name of the moist lesions of the genitals and intertriginous regions, which are rich in spirochetes and highly contagious in secondary syphilis?

Condyloma lata

What is the name of the granulomas that affect the skin and bones in tertiary syphilis?

Gummas

VIRAL PATHOGENS

Which strains of human papillomavirus (HPV) are primarily responsible for genital warts (condylomata acuminata)?

HPV-6 and HPV-11

Pathology Correlate: What is the name of dysplastic cells infected with HPV?

Koilocytes

What virus causes nonpruritic painless 2- to 5-mm umbilicated nodules usually on the trunk and genital area and what is cytoplasmic inclusions examination?

Molluscum contagiosum, a poxvirus, characteristically seen on microscopic

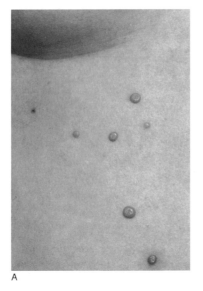
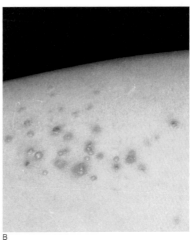

A   B

Figure 51.1   Molluscum contagiosum (note dome shape with central umbilication). (*With permission from Wolff K, Goldsmith L, Katz S, Gilchrest B, Paller A, Leffell D.* Fitzpatrick's Dermatology in General Medicine. *7th ed. New York, NY: McGraw-Hill; 2007.*)

What virus causes recurrent painful vesicular lesions on the genital area and tender inguinal lymphadenopathy?	HSV-2
What virus causes a pruritic rash that consists of macules, papules, vesicles, pustules, and crusty scabs along with fever and malaise typically in school-aged children?	Varicella-zoster virus (chickenpox)
How are the lesions from chickenpox differentiated from smallpox?	For chickenpox, lesions typically occur in different stages simultaneously, have a centripetal distribution (concentrated on the trunk), and are superficial. For smallpox, lesions are all in the same stage, concentrated along the face and extremities, and are described as deep-seated, firm, well-circumscribed.
Name two major, though fortunately rare, complications of varicella zoster virus:	1. Varicella pneumonia (not rare in adults) 2. Encephalitis
What virus causes painful vesicles in a dermatomal distribution?	Varicella-zoster virus (shingles or zoster)

What virus causes vesicular rash on the hands and feet and ulcerations of the mouth?	Coxsackievirus (also known as hand-foot-mouth disease)
What virus causes a bright red facial rash most prominent on the cheeks, a less intense *lacy* rash on the body, and low-grade fevers, runny nose, and sore throat?	Parvovirus B19, erythema infectiosum, also called slapped-cheeks syndrome or fifth disease
What virus causes fever and malaise, progressing to a maculopapular rash extending downward from the face to extremities?	Rubella virus
Why is rubella virus infection concerning in pregnant women?	Rubella virus is one of the TORCH infections and can cause sensorineural deafness, cataracts/glaucoma, cardiac malformations, and neurological problems in the neonate.

FUNGAL PATHOGENS

What systemic fungus in the San Joaquin valley can go to disseminate to almost any organ, but the meninges, bone, and skin are particularly important?	*Coccidioides immitis*
What is erythema nodosum?	Red tender nodules on extensor surfaces (e.g., shins). It is a sign of cell-mediated immunity and commonly occurs after granulomatous diseases such as coccidioidomycosis, tuberculosis, and histoplasmosis. It tends to be a good prognostic factor and is not a sign of disseminated disease.
What is dermatophytosis or tinea?	A pruritic superficial fungal infection caused by several species of dermatophytes
How is it diagnosed?	Visualization of hyphae microscopically in scraping from suspected lesion treated in 10% potassium hydroxide (KOH). The diagnosis may be confirmed by culture.

What dimorphic fungus is typically introduced into the skin by a plant thorn, causing a local pustule or ulcer with nodules along the draining lymphatic?

Sporothrix schenckii

PARASITE PATHOGENS

What parasite causes facial edema and a nodule (chagoma) near the site of the vector bite, coupled with fever, lymphadenopathy, and hepatosplenomegaly during the acute phase of the disease?

Trypanosoma cruzi, Chagas disease. Romaña sign is periorbital edema that occurs in Chagas disease.

What genus of protozoa causes a disease commonly in the Middle East that begins weeks to months after sand fly bites with an initial red papule at the bite site, which enlarges while satellite lesions form and eventually coalesce and ulcerate?

Leishmania

What nematode transmitted by the black fly causes pruritic papules and nodules, a loss of subcutaneous elastin often referred to as *lizard skin*, and eye involvement can cause blindness often referred to as *river blindness*?

Onchocerca volvulus causing onchocerciasis

CHAPTER 52

Musculoskeletal System

SOFT TISSUE INFECTIONS

What species of bacteria commonly infect surgical wounds?

Staphylococcus aureus, Streptococcus, Enterobacter, Pseudomonas aeruginosa, and anaerobes

What species of bacteria commonly infect via traumatic wounds?

Pseudomonas aeruginosa (puncture through shoes) and *Clostridium tetani*

What species of bacteria causes wound infection after cat or dog bites?

Pasteurella multocida

Is osteomyelitis more likely after a cat or dog bite?

Cats have sharper teeth that penetrate periosteum better and directly implant bacteria on bone.

What species of bacteria cause wound infections after human bites besides *Streptococcus* and *Staphylococcus*?

Eikenella corrodens and *Bacteroides*

Should bite wounds be sutured?

No, suturing wounds facilitate anaerobic infections

Which species of bacteria causes gas gangrene?

Clostridium perfringens

How is *C. perfringens* transmitted to result in gas gangrene?

Clostridium perfringens has spores in soil and lives in cells in the colon and vagina. Gas gangrene usually results from traumatic puncture wounds, such as war wounds, motor vehicles accidents, and septic abortion (now rare but was much more common when abortion was illegal).

Why is it called *gas gangrene* and what enzyme is responsible for the unique damage caused by *C. perfringens*?

Enzymes literally digest through tissues, causing accumulation of gas in tissues, myonecrosis, and necrotizing fasciitis. Lecithinase is one of the main enzymes responsible for this damage.

What are some other species of bacteria that cause necrotizing fasciitis?

Streptococcus pyogenes, S. aureus, gram negatives (e.g., *E. coli*), anaerobic bacteria (e.g., *Bacteroides*)

What is the mortality rate for gas gangrene and necrotizing fasciitis?

High (>20%–25%) for both fasciitis and gas gangrene. Death is certain if left untreated.

What is the treatment?

Penicillin G and/or clindamycin, hyperbaric oxygen (bacteriostatic; not always used), wound debridement

What is Fournier gangrene?

Type of necrotizing fasciitis that involves the soft tissue of the male genitalia (often the scrotum), commonly in immunocompromised patients such as diabetics

Which nematode encysts in striated muscle and forms a fibrous capsule that calcifies over years?

Trichinella spiralis

What organisms act as reservoir hosts for *T. spiralis* and how is it transmitted?

Pigs, rats, bears, and seals. Transmission usually occurs through ingestion of raw pork.

How is *T. spiralis* diagnosed?

Muscle biopsy showing larvae encysted within striated muscle

What cestode causes cysticercosis?

Taenia solium (pork tapeworm). *Taenia saginata* (beef tapeworm) does not cause cysticercosis.

What developmental stage of *T. solium* must be ingested to cause cysticercosis?

Eggs must be ingested, usually from fecally contaminated food/water. Ingestion of raw pork does not cause cysticercosis because raw pork contains cysticerci not eggs.

OSTEOMYELITIS

What are common signs and symptoms of osteomyelitis?

Fever, malaise, edema, bone pain (throbbing over affected area), tenderness

How do bacteria usually implant into bone to cause osteomyelitis?

Hematogenous spread from an infected site or direct implantation from a local wound

What is the most common cause of osteomyelitis?

Staphylococcus aureus

What are common causes of osteomyelitis in neonates?

Staphylococcus aureus, enteric gram-negative rods, *Streptococcus agalactiae*

What species of bacteria is a common cause of osteomyelitis in sickle cell anemia patients?

Salmonella. Sickle cell anemia patients are asplenic due to autosplenectomy and cannot clear *Salmonella*.

What species of bacteria is a common cause of osteomyelitis in patients with prosthetic implants?

Staphylococcus epidermidis

What is the most common cause of osteochondritis and osteomyelitis in the foot after a puncture wound through a rubber sole?

Pseudomonas aeruginosa (thrives in the moist environment, due to sweat between layers of the shoe)

What are the special concerns for foot puncture wounds in diabetic patients?

Diabetic patients are more prone to foot puncture wounds because of neuropathy, they are more likely to get osteomyelitis from foot puncture wounds (30%–40%), and they are more likely to get osteomyelitis from direct extension of cellulitis.

What are the findings on radiographic imaging for osteomyelitis?

Lytic focus of bone destruction surrounded by sclerosis

What fungus causes osteomyelitis and is endemic to southwestern United States and Latin America?

Coccidioides immitis (causes valley fever)

What species of zoonotic bacteria enters the body by ingestion of unpasteurized dairy products and frequently causes osteomyelitis?

Brucella species, which cause the disease brucellosis (undulant fever)

What percentage of patients with tuberculosis (TB) has musculoskeletal tuberculosis? What is the most common site of musculoskeletal TB?

1%–3% of all causes of TB. Spine involvement occurs in more than 50% of musculoskeletal tuberculosis (long bones also commonly affected).

What is Pott disease?

Spinal tuberculosis usually involving the lumbar or thoracic vertebrae (characteristically results in kyphosis)

What are the sequelae of Pott disease in severe cases?

Compression fracture of spine, spinal cord, and nerve root compression

ARTHRITIS

How does septic arthritis usually present?

Unilateral acutely swollen, erythematous, painful joint, most commonly the knee (>50%)

What is the overall most common cause of septic arthritis in adults and children older than 2 years?

Staphylococcus aureus

What is the most common cause of septic arthritis in younger, sexually active adults?

Neisseria gonorrhoeae

What species of bacteria is commonly associated with infection in patients with artificial joints?

Staphylococcus epidermidis

What characteristic makes certain strains of *S. epidermidis* more likely to cause infection in patients with artificial joints?

Certain strains produce glycocalyx biofilm and are more likely to adhere to prosthetic surfaces.

What spirochete requires a tick vector and causes arthritis usually in large joints?

Borrelia burgdorferi (Lyme disease). Tick vector is *Ixodes*.

What is the classic finding associated with Lyme disease?

Erythema migrans, raised red rash having well-circumscribed borders that migrate outward from a clear center (typically this clear center is not present), which is the site of the tick bite

How is septic arthritis diagnosed?

Culture, cell count (typically >50,000 neutrophils), and Gram stain of synovial fluid

What species of bacteria causes a postinfection autoimmune disease that commonly damages the heart but can also cause arthritis?

Streptococcus pyogenes. Rheumatic fever can also cause arthritis due to cross-reactivity.

What species of bacteria cause reactive arthritis, a rheumatic arthritis that develops within 1 month following genitourinary or gastrointestinal (GI) infection?

Chlamydia trachomatis, Shigella, Salmonella, Campylobacter jejuni, and *Yersinia enterocolitica*

What genetic subtype makes patients more susceptible to reactive arthritis?

Human leukocyte antigen (HLA)-B27

What is reactive arthritis (Reiter syndrome)?

Clinical triad of uveitis, urethritis, and arthritis

What viruses can cause arthritis secondary to immune complex crossover?

Parvovirus B19, rubella, and hepatitis B virus Mnemonic: Can't see, can't pee, can't climb a tree.

Index

Note: Page numbers followed by *f* indicate figures and *t* indicate tables.